Non-Hodgkin's Lymphomas in Children

Non-Hodgkin's Lymphomas in Children

edited by

John Graham-Pole, M.D., M.R.C.P.
Associate Professor of Pediatrics
Division of Hematology/Oncology
Rainbow Babies and Childrens Hospital
Cleveland, Ohio

MASSON Publishing USA, Inc.

New York • Paris • Barcelona • Milan • Mexico City • Rio de Janeiro

ISBN 0-89352-068-3

Library of Congress Catalog Card Number: 80-81990

Printed in the United States of America

Masson Monographs in Pediatric Hematology/Oncology

Carl Pochedly, M.D. and Denis R. Miller, M.D.
Series Editors

Transfusion Therapy: The Fetus, Infant, and Child (1980)
edited by William C. Sherwood, M.D. and Alan Cohen, M.D.

Non-Hodgkin's Lymphomas in Children (1980)
edited by John Graham-Pole, M.D.

PREFACE

In the last two decades, enormous strides have been made in our understanding of the biologic behavior of many childhood cancers. Many of these diseases can now be cured. Indeed, about one-half of affected children enjoy the prospect of a normal life span. However, pediatric oncology still poses numerous perplexing questions.

Non-Hodgkin's lymphoma presents a particular challenge to oncologists. Wide variations in its pathologic appearances, surface antigenic expression, clinical manifestations, and prognosis emphasize the heterogeneous nature of this group of disorders. It has distinct characteristics not shared by its adult counterpart. In all, it accounts for nearly 10% of childhood cancers.

"Total therapy," so successfully employed in the treatment of acute lymphoblastic leukemia in children, has in recent years been applied to non-Hodgkin's lymphoma, but, of necessity, with even greater intensity. The result has been significantly improved long-term control of this notoriously resistant disease — although often at the price of severe toxicity. Fortunately we can now identify histologic and immunologic subsets of lymphoma and can plan more selective treatment strategies. The hoped-for outcome, of course, is treatment that achieves an increasing cure rate at a much lower level of toxicity to the patient.

In this monograph, I have brought together clinicians and basic scientists who have already made important contributions to our understanding of critical aspects of this disease: its etiology, pathology, immunology, diagnosis, treatment, and specific complications. I have solicited contributions from both American and British workers, to bring a measure of both balance and controversy to the pages of this text. It is not intended as a comprehensive treatise, but rather, as a concise, up-to-date volume that will appeal to all whose work brings them either continuously or infrequently into contact with children with cancer.

CONTRIBUTORS

Costan W. Berard, MD
Chief, Hematopathology Section
Laboratory of Pathology
National Institutes of Health
Bethesda, MD

Jeffrey Cossman, MD
Senior Investigator, Hematopathology Section
Laboratory of Pathology
National Institutes of Health
Bethesda, MD
Instructor, Department of Pathology
University of Michigan Medical School
Ann Arbor, MI

John E. Freeman, MRCP, FRCR
Clinical Professor of Radiology
University of Texas Health Sciences Center
San Antonio, TX

John Graham-Pole, MD, MRCP
Associate Professor of Pediatrics
School of Medicine
Case Western Reserve University
Cleveland, OH
Division of Hematology/Oncology
Rainbow Babies and Childrens Hospital
Cleveland, OH

J. A. Habeshaw, PhD, MD
Senior Scientific Officer
Imperial Cancer Research Fund
Department of Medical Oncology
St. Batholomew's Hospital
London, England

Herbert Kaizer, MD, PhD
Assistant Professor of Oncology and Pediatrics
The Oncology Center
Department of Pediatrics
The Johns Hopkins University
School of Medicine
Baltimore, MD

Elizabeth Kurczynski, MD
Assistant Professor of Pediatrics
School of Medicine
Case Western Reserve University
Cleveland, OH

Brigid G. Leventhal, MD
Director of Pediatric Oncology
Associate Professor of Oncology and Pediatrics
The Oncology Center
Department of Pediatrics
The Johns Hopkins University
School of Medicine
Baltimore, MD

Anna T. Meadows, MD
Associate Physician
Division of Oncology
The Children's Hospital of Philadelphia
Philadelphia, PA

Martin Mott, MB, MRCP
Consultant Paediatric Oncologist
Department of Child Health
Royal Hospital for Sick Children
Bristol, England

Margaret P. Sullivan, MD
Pediatrician
M. D. Anderson Hospital and Tumor Institute
Professor of Pediatrics
The University of Texas Cancer System
Houston, TX

Adrian R. Timothy, MRCP, FRCR
Consultant in Radiotherapy and Oncology
St. Thomas Hospital
London, England

Stuart R. Toledano, MD
Assistant Physician
Division of Oncology
The Children's Hospital of Philadelphia
Philadelphia, PA

Michael Willoughby, MD
Consultant Haematologist
Department of Paediatric Haematology/Oncology
Royal Hospital for Sick Children
Glasgow, Scotland
Lecturer in Paediatric Haematology
Faculty of Medicine
University of Glasgow
Glasgow, Scotland

John L. Ziegler, MD
Associate Director
Clinical Oncology Program
Division of Cancer Treatment
National Cancer Institute

CONTENTS

PREFACE vii
CONTRIBUTORS ix

CHAPTER 1 1

Etiologic Factors in Non-Hodgkin's Lymphoma

B. G. Leventhal and H. Kaizer

CHAPTER 2 13

Histopathology of Childhood Non-Hodgkin's Lymphomas

J. Cossman and C. W. Berard

CHAPTER 3 37

Investigation of Non-Hodgkin's Lymphoma in Children by Surface Phenotyping Techniques

J. A. Habeshaw

CHAPTER 4 63

Diagnosis and Staging of Non-Hodgkin's Lymphoma in Childhood

S. R. Toledano and A. T. Meadows

CHAPTER 5 81

Chemotherapy of Childhood Non-Hodgkin's Lymphoma

M. Mott

CHAPTER 6 95

Treatment of Non-Hodgkin's Lymphomas: Radiotherapy

A. R. Timothy and J. E. Freeman

CHAPTER 7 107

Mass and Metabolic Effects of Non-Hodgkin's Lymphomas in Children

E. Kurczynski and J. Graham-Pole

CHAPTER 8 131

Burkitt's Lymphoma

J. L. Ziegler

CHAPTER 9 147

Bone Marrow and CNS Involvement in Non-Hodgkin's Lymphoma

M. Willoughby

CHAPTER 10 165

Non-Hodgkin's Lymphomas in Children: An Overview

M. P. Sullivan

Index 173

CHAPTER ONE

Etiologic Factors in Non-Hodgkin's Lymphoma

BRIGID G. LEVENTHAL, MD; HERBERT KAIZER, MD, PhD

NON-HODGKIN'S LYMPHOMA is a polymorphic disorder. The morphologic and functional subclassifications of this disease are discussed in other chapters of this book (see chapters 2 and 4). For the purposes of our present discussion, it is sufficient to note that the majority of cases of non-Hodgkin's lymphoma have been shown to have either B or T markers,[1,2] or both,[3] while only a few have been found to lack these markers.[4] This is important because it implies that lymphoma cells usually resemble functionally differentiated normal cells, as opposed to the cells of childhood acute lymphocytic leukemia, which usually resemble more primitive "null" cells. In addition, it should be noted that the majority of lymphomas that have been cytologically analyzed have been shown to have a monoclonal origin.[5] However, the recently described variant of lymphoma, immunoblastic sarcoma,[6] appears to have its origin in a condition called immunoblastic lymphadenopathy, which can begin as a polyclonal B-cell proliferation.

The etiology of non-Hodgkin's lymphoma is probably complex and multifactorial. On the one hand, therefore, our discussion will include numerous potential etiologic factors such as viruses, cytogenetic abnormalities, and immunodeficiency states. On the other hand, a unifying thread in this chapter is the emphasis on recent observations suggesting that some non-Hodgkin's lymphomas represent complex examples of an immune response gone awry.

RNA VIRUSES

Type-C RNA viruses are found in many mammalian species; in mice they are consistently found in both inbred and wild strains. Although certain virus isolates

---

The Oncology Center, Department of Pediatrics, The Johns Hopkins University, School of Medicine, 601 N. Broadway, Baltimore, MD 21205

are not associated with demonstrable oncogenic activity,[7] many are clearly associated with leukemogenesis and lymphomagenesis.[8] Oncogenicity by these viruses can occur by either vertical (germ cell) or horizontal (post-conception) transmission.

In the vertically transmitted or endogenous virus, the genome is integrated at specific chromosomal loci.[9] Spontaneous onset of endogenous virus replication occurs at different times in different inbred strains, and thus the latent period for tumor induction varies with each virus type and is also influenced by genetic and constitutional factors.[7] Endogenous viral replication, and presumably lymphomagenesis as well, can also be initiated after exposure of the cell to agents such as irradiation, chemicals, or even exogenous viruses.[8]

Exogenous viruses are usually integrated at sites in DNA that are not specific.[8] Exogenous viruses have been shown to cause malignancies that are horizontally transmitted, notably cat[10] and bovine leukemia and lymphoma.[11] In these situations constitutional factors can be shown to play a role. Older cats, for example, are less susceptible to infection than neonates.[10] In addition, it should be noted that both feline and bovine leukemias may be controlled by prophylactic immunization.[12,13]

Thus there is convincing evidence for both vertical and horizontal transmission of lymphatic leukemia and lymphoma associated with type-C RNA viruses in animals. The techniques for detecting similar viruses in human tumors, such as the isolation of reverse transcriptase from cells, have been available for some years. Nevertheless, definitive identification of human RNA tumor viruses has not yet been achieved. Serologic evidence for the occurrence of primate C-type virus in humans is also ambiguous.[7] Although occasional viruses have been isolated from human leukemic material, there is no evidence that such viruses are consistently present; nor is there any evidence that the complete viral genomes of the virus isolates are present in the patients from whom they are isolated.[14]

DNA VIRUSES

There are many types of DNA viruses that have been shown to cause malignant transformation of cells in tissue culture, as well as producing tumors in experimental animals.[15] The class of virus most frequently associated with naturally occurring tumors has been the herpes viruses. Marek's disease of chickens is an example of a lymphoproliferative disorder caused by a horizontally transmitted herpes-type virus.[16] Evidence for horizontal transmission and immunological control of the disorder was substantiated by the success of a program of prophylactic vaccination.[17] There is good evidence that Marek's disease is a T-cell neoplasm.[16] This disease is also under genetic control in that the major histocompatibility gene B^{21} is associated with resistance to Marek's disease.[18] At least three simian herpes viruses have been isolated that cause non-Hodgkin's lymphoma in some nonhuman primate species. These viruses have been reviewed by Deinhardt,[19] who commented on their similarities to EB virus. This latter virus has been shown to cause lymphoma in New World monkeys.[20]

The DNA virus that is most clearly associated with human malignant lymphomas is the Epstein-Barr (EB) virus. This virus is implicated clinically in the development of infectious mononucleosis as well as in African Burkitt's lymphoma and lymphoepithelioma. Infection of lymphoid cells with EB virus *in vitro* can transform them into long-term tissue culture cell lines. The transformed state is always associated with detectable EB nuclear antigen (EBNA).[21] In infectious mononucleosis in normal individuals, it is felt that the EB virus infects the B-cells, which undergo proliferation. Within a few weeks, however, cytotoxic T-cells predominate among the atypical lymphocytes in the peripheral blood.[22,23] It is postulated that these T-cells are responding to EB viral antigens on the B-cells and destroy the transformed B-cells as they proliferate.

It is postulated that uncontrolled proliferation of B-cells, which have been neoplastically transformed by EB virus, is an important factor in the development of Burkitt's lymphoma. Burkitt's lymphoma is endemic in Africa in areas where malaria is also endemic. EB virus has been isolated from biopsy specimens and from long-term tissue culture cell lines from patients with Burkitt's lymphoma.[24] In addition, almost all of the African tumors contain EB viral genome DNA[25] and EB nuclear antigen (EBNA).[21] Burkitt's lymphoma also arises sporadically in other parts of the world, including the United States. About 80% of the American cases, however, are not associated with the Epstein-Barr virus. Thus no viral DNA-positive or EBNA-positive cells are detected in the tumors, and the patients have antibody profiles comparable to those of normal children. The remaining 20% of the American cases of Burkitt's lymphoma are associated with the EB virus and are indistinguishable from their African counterparts, except that in the United States the age range of the patients is shifted toward adolescence and young adulthood.[26]

Thus it is clear that the EB virus has the capacity to transform lymphocytes. However, not all cases of Burkitt's lymphoma are associated with EB virus infection, and only a small fraction of individuals infected with EB virus develop Burkitt's lymphoma. It has been proposed that perhaps in areas where early infection with this virus and Burkitt's lymphoma are endemic, the tumor occurs only in patients with some abnormal degree of response to the EB virus. Possibly this abnormal response to the EB virus is conditioned by the state of their concurrent malaria. Serologic screening of over 45,000 African children who were then followed clinically showed that those 14 who later developed Burkitt's lymphoma had an unusually high antibody titer to viral capsid antigen (VCA). These data were interpreted as showing that a heavy, persistent viral carrier state predisposed children to Burkitt's lymphoma, although additional factors were required for the development of the tumor.[26,27]

GENETIC FACTORS

The study of tumor karyotypes with the aid of chromosome banding has revealed preferential involvement of certain chromosomes in non-Hodgkin's lymphoma. A consistent translocation onto the long arm (q) of one chromosome in the number 14 chromosome pair was first noted in African Burkitt's lymphoma by Manolov and Manolova.[28] In several cell lines from African and North America Burkitt's lymphoma, this translocation has been shown to be material from the long arm of chromosome 8.[29,30]

Chromosome 14 abnormalities have also been implicated in other lymphoid neoplasms, particularly those of B-cell origin.[30] Fleischman and Prigogina[32] reported at least two cases with translocation of material from the long arm of chromosome 11 to the long arm of chromosome 14. In addition, chromosome abnormalities, frequently involving the chromosome 14 pair, have been revealed in lymphocytes from patients with ataxia telangiectasia. Gradual rise of a single aberrant clone during the course of disease, and development of chronic lymphoid leukemia from this clone with tandem translocation 14q:14q, has been reported by McCaw *et al.*[33] These abnormalities of chromosome 14 appear to be associated specifically with lymphoma and not with infection of the cell by EB virus.[30] It is the feeling of McCaw and coworkers [30] that abnormalities of chromosome 14 in lymphoma parallel those of the Philadelphia (Ph^1) chromosome seen in chronic myeloid leukemia. The 14q+ translocation may represent a comparable tissue-specific nonrandom characteristic of lymphocytic neoplasia.

The mechanism by which balanced translocations affect normal cell growth and differentiation has not yet been elucidated, although once they occur they may result in a cell that is unusually susceptible to malignant transformation by EB virus. Alternatively, Klein[21] has postulated that Burkitt's lymphoma develops in at least three steps. The first step is the EB-virus-induced immortalization of some B lymphocytes upon primary infection. The second step is brought about by an environment-dependent factor, perhaps chronic holoendemic malaria. This would stimulate the latent EB-virus-carrying cells, frozen at a particular stage of B-cell differentiation, to chronic proliferation. By forcing the long-lived preneoplastic cells to repeated division, the environmental cofactor would provide the scenario for cytogenetic diversification. The third and final step would take place if and when the "right" translocation occurred on chromosome 14, which would lead to the outgrowth of an autonomous monoclonal tumor. It has been observed that chromosome 14 is frequently involved in the genesis of human neoplasia of largely, if not exclusively, B-cell origin. According to Klein,[21] this finding suggests that some determinant(s) on chromosome 14 are closely involved with the normal responsiveness of the B lymphocyte to growth-controlling mechanisms.

GENETICALLY DETERMINED IMMUNODEFICIENCY DISEASES (GDID)

It is well known that several congenital immunodeficiency diseases are associated with a high risk of malignancy. Data from the Immunodeficiency Cancer Registry have recently been published.[34] The diseases most frequently associated with malignancy per patient seen with this diagnosis by the group of reporting physicians are as follows: Wiskott-Aldrich syndrome, 21 out of 136 (15.4%); ataxia telangiectasia, 33 out of 283 (11.7%); selective decrease/absence of IgM, 8 out of 79 (10%); and combined variable immunodeficiency disease with onset over age 16 years, 18 out of 211 (8.5%). Malignancy occurred less commonly in other subcategories of immunodeficiency disease. It is of interest that in X-linked (Bruton's) hypogammaglobulinemia, where the incidence of leukemia was once thought to be high, this survey showed cancer in only 2 out of 274 patients (0.7%).

The general malignancy patterns observed in these data include the following. If a child with genetically determined immunodeficiency disease develops a malignancy, it will most often be a non-Hodgkin's lymphoma. If an adult with GDID develops a malignancy, it will be non-Hodgkin's lymphoma or carcinoma in approximately equal proportions. The most common single histologic type of non-Hodgkin's lymphoma in the registry is histiocytic lymphoma. Phenotypic characteristics of a small series of lymphoreticular tumors from patients with genetically determined immunodeficiency disease indicate that malignant blast cells are usually B- or T-like in origin, rather than "null" cell (non-T, non-B).

Louie and Schwartz[31] recently reviewed the relationship of immunodeficiency and cancer. They point out that the genetic disorders which are commonly associated with malignancy, including those cited above and Bloom's syndrome, are associated with multiple abnormalities outside the immune system. Thus both the immunodeficiency and the malignancy may represent different manifestations of a single underlying disorder, rather than the malignancy being a consequence of the immunodeficiency. Genetic disturbance in these conditions can manifest itself by structural changes in chromosomes. All of these disorders are associated with increased frequency of DNA damage, which has been interpreted as a failure of DNA repair after injury.[35,36] This, however, does not explain why the preponderance of malignancies in patients with congenital immunodeficiency comprises lymphomas and leukemias.

The most common neoplasms of children are acute lymphoblastic leukemia, brain tumors, neuroblastoma, and Wilms' tumor; however, none of these tumors has an increased frequency in these children. Thus the shift toward lymphoma in these diseases seems real. Louie and Schwartz[31] feel that the explanation may lie in the tendency of cells with high mitotic indices to accumulate mutations. If there is chromosome instability to begin with, the risk of new mutations may be considerably increased in frequently dividing cells. In support of this theory, they note that the second most common malignancy in Bloom's syndrome and ataxia telangiectasia involves the gastrointestinal tract.

DUNCAN'S DISEASE

Another possible explanation for the occurrence of a high incidence of lymphomas in patients with immunodeficiency might involve an abnormal susceptibility to infection with an "oncogenic" virus. Purtilo *et al.*[37] in 1975 described a family in which 6 out of 18 male cousins died of a lymphoproliferative disease. These cases exhibited a subtle progressive combined variable immunodeficiency disease characterized by benign or malignant proliferation of lymphocytes and alteration in the concentrations of serum immunoglobulins ranging from agammaglobulinemia to polyclonal hyperglobulinemia. Infectious mononucleosis occurred during or preceding terminal events in at least three of the cousins. This study suggested that, in this family, the EB virus or other viruses triggered a fatal proliferation of lymphocytes and that progressive attrition of T-cell function allowed uncontrolled proliferation of B-cells, resulting in documented lymphoma in at least two of the cases.[23] This then might be considered a familial immunodeficiency disorder that is expressed only on exposure to EB virus. It is of interest that several of these boys had clinically normal courses of other childhood infections including varicella prior to the onset of their terminal disease.

Joncas *et al.*[38] have reported a relatively high incidence of EB virus early antigen in the serum of patients with ataxia telangiectasia. This finding suggests that EB virus, as well as the abnormal chromosomes, may play a role in the malignant transformation of cells from these patients.

DISEASE ASSOCIATED WITH MANIPULATION OF THE IMMUNE SYSTEM

Renal transplantation

It has been known for some time that the risk of developing malignant tumors is greatly increased in recipients of renal allografts.[39] A disproportionate number of neoplasms that develop in these patients are lymphomas. The most common type of lymphoma in transplant recipients is often termed reticulum cell sarcoma or histiocytic lymphoma. Closer analysis, however, reveals that many of these cases may in fact fit into the category of immunoblastic sarcoma.[6]

It has been postulated that the malignancies which develop in these individuals are a consequence of the immunosuppressive therapy used in the posttransplant period. Louie and Schwartz[31] again caution us against the acceptance of an overall defect in immune surveillance as an explanation for this phenomenon. They point out that a faulty tumor surveillance mechanism, with lack of recognition of tumor neoantigens, should not favor one particular form of cancer over another. However, lymphomas are highly prevalent in this group, and the more common tumors, such as carcinoma of the lung and breast, are rarely seen in patients who have received immunosuppressive therapy. Second, the actual extent of immunologic impairment in recipients of organ transplants who develop neoplasms is unknown. Many patients treated with azathioprine, with or without prednisone, respond normally to antigenic stimuli,[40] and many allograft recipients who develop a tumor have suffered repeated rejection crises, indicating a relatively intact immune system.[41]

However, it is quite conceivable that immunosuppressive therapy might alter the immune response to infectious agents in a way that would favor the development of malignancy. Ascher *et al.* (cited in ref. 31) report a 19-year-old renal allograft recipient who developed immunoblastic sarcoma several weeks after exposure to infectious mononucleosis. They postulate that this patient's T-cells could not eliminate EB-virus-infected B-cells in the usual manner, thus permitting development of the tumor. Here again one can postulate that immunosuppressive therapy resulted in selective defects in immunoregulation that allowed uncontrolled proliferation, not of all malignant clones, but rather of selected clones of cells from within the immune system.

Thymic transplantation

Borzy *et al.*[42] have reported three cases of fatal lymphoma after transplantation of cultured thymus in children with combined immunodeficiency disease. Each of these patients received an intraperitoneal transplant of cultured thymus and developed a fatal polyclonal B-cell immunoblastic lymphoproliferative disorder shortly after transplantation. Their series included 30 patients who had various immunodeficiency diseases and had received 50 separate transplants, making the incidence of this disorder 3 out of 30, or about 10%. This rate does not exceed the incidence of malignant immunoblastic disease reported to occur in patients with selective IgM deficiency in the Immunodeficiency Malignancy Registry. It is, therefore, possible that these patients would have developed this type of process in any case. The authors of this report point out, on the other hand, that it is possible that the cultured thymus transplant could have acted as a promoter, causing an uncontrolled polyclonal immunoblastic B-cell proliferation in patients without sufficient control mechanisms.

AUTOIMMUNE DISEASE

Autoimmune hemolytic anemia is frequently associated with lymphoma, but will not be discussed here since it is not known which disorder is primary and which is secondary. It has been known for many years that patients with Sjögren's syndrome develop pseudolymphoma and frank non-Hodgkin's lymphoma as part of the natural history of their disease.[43] Patients with systemic lupus erythematosus (SLE) also have been noted to have an increased incidence of malignancy, even those not receiving immunosuppressive therapy.[31] In several cases of autoimmune disease, the process which has developed is that which is now called immunoblastic lymphadenopathy or immunoblastic sarcoma.[6]

In New Zealand black (NZB) mice, a strain that suffers from congenital autoimmune disorders which terminate in malignant lymphoma, aging has been shown to be associated with a deficiency of suppressor T-cell function. It has been postulated that this deficiency allows unbridled proliferation of B lymphocytes. There is good evidence in SLE for the occurrence of unregulated B-cell activity leading to production of antibodies to suppressor T-cells and dysfunction of suppressor T-cell mechanisms.[45] Defective immune regulation can again be held responsible for allowing chronic unsuppressed antigenic stimulation, leading to benign or "premalignant" polyclonal proliferation and subsequent monoclonal lymphoid malignancy. This mechanism may be important in lymphomagenesis.

CHRONIC ANTIGENIC STIMULATION

It is evident from the foregoing that chronic unregulated antigenic stimulation may be an important pathogenic factor in the development of lymphomas, both in those lymphomas induced by viruses and in those associated with autoimmune diseases. There is evidence for this mechanism from other sources also. Metcalf[46] repeatedly injected *Salmonella adelaide* vaccine or bovine serum albumin into mice, and observed an increased incidence of sarcoma and plasma cell tumors. Immunoblastic lymphoma with mixed cryoglobulinemia has been reported[47] in one patient who had received liver extract by injection and by mouth for many years. The investigators felt the disorder was related to the chronic antigenic stimulation. The lymphoma and cryoglobulinemia regressed following removal of the antigen and the administration of one course of chemotherapy with cyclophosphamide, vincristine, and prednisone.

In their description of immunoblastic lymphadenopathy, Lukes and Tindle[6] observe that the signs and symptoms of the disorder occurred with dramatic onset after administration of therapeutic agents for a variety of conditions in 6 out of 22 patients (27%). These therapeutic agents included penicillin in four cases, griseofulvin in one, and diphenylhydantoin in one. Diphenylhydantoin has long been associated with abnormal lymphoid proliferation, although an immune basis for this has not been proven. Chronic stimulation by tissue antigens was thought by Schwartz and Beldotti[48] to be a possible etiologic factor in the lymphomas they observed in mice that were long-term survivors of graft-vs.-host reactions. However, these tumors eventually proved to be of recipient origin. Gossett *et al.*[49] have recently reported a case of an immunoblastic sarcoma that occurred in donor cells after bone marrow transplantation. This patient had moderately severe graft-vs.-host disease. The authors did not exclude the possible etiologic contributions of immunodeficiency, therapy, and occult viral infections. However, they felt that the stimulus for B-cell proliferation had most probably been provided by the chronic antigenic stimulation that resulted from antigenic incompatibility between donor and recipient.

SUMMARY

The majority of cases of non-Hodgkin's lymphoma demonstrate the presence of specific immunologic markers; in other words, they are B, T, or double marker cells. In the last few years, observations that have potential etiologic import have been made most consistently in the area of B-cell tumors. It appears that there may well be a spectrum of disorders which range from polyclonal immunoblastic lymphadenopathy to monoclonal Burkitt's lymphoma. This concept forces us to place new emphasis, in explaining etiology, on the regulatory interactions within the immune system. The breakdown of the normal regulatory system could result either from the production of B cells, which have a selective growth advantage, such as through transformation by EB virus, through the 14q+ translocation, or from controller cells that have been inactivated, perhaps genetically or through the use of drugs.

Chronic antigenic stimulation leading to unchecked lymphoid proliferation may be an etiologic factor common to hereditary and acquired immunodeficiency disease, oncogenic viral infections, and autoimmune disease. In all the examples that have recently been described, it appears that more than one factor has been simultaneously operative.

ACKNOWLEDGMENT

This work was supported in part by Grant CA-06973-16 from the National Cancer Institute, DHEW.

References

1. Murphy SB, Melvin SL, Mauer AM: Correlation of tumor cell kinetic studies with surface marker results in childhood non-Hodgkin's lymphoma. *Cancer Res 39:1534, 1979.*
2. Mann RB, Jaffe ES, Berard CW: Malignant lymphomas; a conceptual understanding of morphologic diversity. *Am J Pathol 94:105, 1979.*
3. Coccia PF, Kersey JH, Corte J, *et al*: Lymphoblasts with receptors for both erythrocytes and complement in childhood diffuse poorly differentiated lymphocytic lymphoma (dPDLL). *Blood 46:1036, 1975.*
4. Jaffe EF, Braylan RC, Frank MM, *et al*: Heterogeneity of immunologic markers and surface morphology in childhood lymphoblastic lymphoma. *Blood 48:213, 1976.*
5. Friedman JM, Fialkow PH: Cell marker studies of human tumorigenesis. *Transplant Rev 28:17, 1976.*
6. Lukes RJ, Tindle BH: Immunoblastic lymphadenopathy; a hyperimmune entity resembling Hodgkin's disease. *N Engl. J Med 292:1, 1975.*
7. Ihle JN: Experimental models and conceptual approaches to studies of lymphomas and leukemia; etiology, biology, and control. *Semin Hematol 15:95, 1978.*
8. Kaplan HS: Etiology of lymphomas and leukemias; role of C-type RNA virus. *Leukemia Res 2:253, 1978.*
9. Chattopadhyay SK, Rowe WP, Teich NM, Lowy DR: Definite evidence that the murine C-type virus inducing locus AKV-1 is viral genetic material. *Proc Natl Acad Sci USA 72:906, 1975.*
10. Essex M. Cotter SM, Sliski AH, *et al*: Horizontal transmission of feline leukemia virus under natural conditions in a feline leukemia cluster household. *Int J Cancer 19:90, 1977.*
11. Burny A, Bex F, Chantrenne H, *et al*: Bovine leukemia virus involvement in enzootic bovine leukosis. *Adv Cancer Res 28:251, 1978.*
12. Jarrett W, Jarrett O, Mackey L, *et al*: Vaccination against feline leukemia virus using a cell membrane antigen system. *Int J Cancer 16:134, 1975.*
13. Olsen RG, Hoover EA, Mathes LE, *et al*: Immunization against feline oncornavirus disease using a killed tumor cell vaccine. *Cancer Res 36:3642, 1976.*
14. Reitz MS, Miller NR, Wong-Staal F, *et al*: Primate type-C virus nucleic acid sequences (woolly monkey and baboon types) in tissues from a patient with acute myelogenous leukemia and in viruses isolated from cultured cells of the same patient. *Proc Natl Acad Sci USA 73:2113, 1976.*
15. Rapp F, Westmoreland D: Cell transformation by DNA containing viruses. *Biochim Biophys Acta 458:167, 1976.*
16. Payne LN: Viral lymphomagenesis in the domestic fowl; a review. *Proc Roy Soc Med 70:559, 1977.*

17. Lesnik F, Ross LJN: Immunization against Marek's disease using Marek's disease virus-specific antigens free from infectious virus. *Int J Cancer 16:153, 1975.*
18. Longenecker BM, Pazderka, F, Gavora JS, *et al*: Role of the major histocompatibility complex in resistance to Marek's disease; restriction of the growth of JMV-MD tumor cells in genetically resistant birds. *Adv Exp Med Biol 88:287, 1977.*
19. Deinhardt F: Virus induced lymphoproliferative disease in non-human primates. *Br J Cancer 31 (suppl II):140, 1975.*
20. Frank A, Andeman WA, Miller G: The Epstein-Barr virus and nonhuman primates; natural and experimental infection. *Adv Cancer Res 23:171, 1976.*
21. Klein G: Lymphoma development in mice and humans; diversity of initiation is followed by convergent cytogenetic evolution. *Proc Natl Acad Sci USA 76:2442, 1979.*
22. Denman AM, Pelton BK: Control mechanisms in infectious mononucleosis. *Clin Exp Immunol 18:13, 1974.*
23. Mangi RJ, Neiderman JC, Kelleher JE, *et al*: Depression in all cell-mediated immunity during acute infectious mononucleosis. *N Engl J Med 291:1149–1153, 1974.*
24. Epstein MA, Achong BG, Barr YM: Virus particles in cultured lymphoblasts from Burkitt's lymphoma. *Lancet 1:702, 1964.*
25. Zur Hausen H, Schulte-Holthausen H, Klein G, *et al*: EBV DNA in biopsies of Burkitt's tumours and anaplastic carcinomas of the nasopharynx. *Nature 228:1056, 1970.*
26. Henle W, Henle G, Lennette ET: The Epstein Barr virus. *Sci. Am. 241(1):48, 1979.*
27. De The G, Geser A, Day NE, *et al*: Epidemiologic evidence for causal relationship between Epstein-Barr virus and Burkitt's lymphoma from Ugandan prospective study. *Nature (London) 274:756, 1978.*
28. Manolov G, Manolova Y: Marker band in one chromosome 14 from Burkitt lymphomas. *Nature (London) 237:33, 1972.*
29. Zech L, Haglund U, Nilsson K, *et al*: Characteristic chromosomal abnormalities in biopsies and lymphoid cell lines from patients with Burkitt and non-Burkitt lymphomas. *Int J Cancer 17:47, 1976.*
30. McCaw BK, Epstein AL, Kaplan HS, *et al*: Chromosome 14 translocation in African and North American Burkitt's lymphoma. *Int J Cancer 19:482, 1977.*
31. Louie S, Schwartz RS: Immunodeficiency and the pathogenesis of lymphoma and leukemia. *Semin Hematol 15:117, 1978.*
32. Fleischman EW, Prigogina EL: Karyotype pecularities of malignant lymphomas. *Hum Genet 35:269, 1977.*
33. McCaw KB, Hecht F, Harnden DG, *et al*: Somatic rearrangement of chromosome 14 in human lymphocytes. *Proc Natl Acad Sci USA 72:2071, 1975.*
34. Spector BD, Perry GS, Kersey JH: Genetically determined immunodeficiency diseases (GDID) and malignancy; report from the Immunodeficiency-Cancer Registry. *Clin Immunol Immunopathol 11:12, 1978.*
35. Taylor AMR, Metcalfe JA, Oxford JM, *et al*: Is chromatid type damage in ataxia telangiectasia after irradiation at G_0 a consequence of defective repair? *Nature 260:441, 1976.*
36. Gianelli F, Benson PF, Pawsey SA, *et al*: Ultraviolet light sensitivity and delayed DNA chain maturation in Bloom's syndrome fibroblasts. *Nature 265:466, 1977.*
37. Purtilo DT, Cassel CK, Yang JPS, *et al*: X-linked recessive progressive combined variable immunodeficiency (Duncan's disease) *Lancet 1:935, 1975.*
38. Joncas J, Lapointe N, Gervais F: Unusual prevalence of antibodies to Epstein-Barr virus early antigen in ataxia telangiectasia. *Lancet 2:1160, 1977.*
39. Penn I: Malignancies associated with the renal transplantation. *Urology 10:52(suppl), 1977.*
40. Swanson M, Schwartz RS: Immunosuppressive therapy; the relation between clinical response and immunologic competence. *N Engl J Med 277:163, 1967.*
41. McKhann CF: Primary malignancy in patients undergoing immunosuppression for renal transplantation. *Transplantation 8:209, 1969.*

42. Borzy MS, Hong R, Horowitz SD, *et al*: Fatal lymphoma after transplantation of cultured thymus in children with combined immunodeficiency disease. *N Engl J Med 301:565, 1979.*
43. Roubinian JR, Talal N: Neoplasia, autoimmunity and the immune response. *Adv Intern Med 23:435, 1978.*
44. Waldmann TA, Blaese RM, Broder S, *et al*: Disorders of suppressor immunoregulatory cells in the pathogenesis of immunodeficiency and autoimmunity. *Ann Intern Med 88:226, 1978.*
45. Raveche ES, Steinberg AD: Lymphocytes and lymphocyte function in SLE. *Semin Hematol 16:344, 1979.*
46. Metcalf D: Reticular tumors in mice subjected to prolonged antigenic stimulation. *Br J Cancer 15:769, 1961.*
47. Schultz DR, Yunis AA: Immunoblastic lymphadenopathy with mixed cryoglobulinemia; a detailed case study. *N Engl J Med 292:8, 1975.*
48. Schwartz RS, Beldotti L: Malignant lymphomas following allogenic disease; transition from an immunological to a neoplastic disorder. *Science 149:1511, 1965.*
49. Gossett TC, Gale RP, Fleischman H, *et al*: Immunoblastic sarcoma in donor cells after bone marrow transplantation. *N Engl J Med 300:904, 1979.*

CHAPTER TWO

Histopathology of Childhood Non-Hodgkin's Lymphomas

JEFFREY COSSMAN, MD; COSTAN W. BERARD, MD

IN THE UNITED STATES, leukemias (30–35%) and malignant lymphomas (5–10%) account together for almost 50% of all cancers in patients under 15 years of age.[1] The precise relative figures are difficult to establish because it is not always possible to draw sharp distinctions between acute leukemia and non-Hodgkin's lymphomas in children. Both Hodgkin's disease and non-Hodgkin's lymphomas occur over a broad age range in children. Hodgkin's disease comprises about 40% of childhood lymphomas, is rare below 5 years of age, and increases in frequency from ages 5 to 15. Non-Hodgkin's lymphomas occur more frequently than Hodgkin's disease in patients under five years of age. They, too, however, are seen predominantly in children 5 to 15 years old and comprise about 60% of childhood lymphomas. In children, non-Hodgkin's lymphomas show a male preponderance with sex ratios (male:female) in the range of 2–3:1.

Compared to the leukemias and lymphomas, other pediatric tumors occur with the following frequencies: CNS tumors, 16–18%; neuroblastoma, 7–9%; Wilms' tumor, 5–8%; bone sarcomas (mostly osteogenic and Ewing's), 4–5%; rhabdomyosarcoma, 2–3%; and retinoblastoma, 1–2%.[2] Children clearly have a predilection for reticuloendothelial neoplasms, sarcomas, and embryonal tumors (Wilms' tumor, retinoblastoma, neuroblastoma). Carcinomas comprise only 5% of pediatric cancers. These figures are in marked contrast to those of the general adult population, in which the cancer incidence is as follows: carcinomas, 85%; leukemia-lymphoma, 6%; sarcomas, 3%; and embryonal tumors, 1%.[1] Confronted with a poorly differentiated malignant tumor in a child, the surgical pathologist should strongly suspect a mesenchymal or lymphoid rather than an epithelial origin for the neoplasm.

Laboratory of Pathology, National Institutes of Health, Bethesda, MD 20014

CLASSIFICATION

Histopathologists traditionally have classified malignant lymphomas descriptively according to morphologic observations. However, recent advances in the identification of immunologic surface markers and enzyme cytochemistry have markedly refined our understanding of the lymphomas and have established them as neoplasms of the immune system. Such advances have been particularly apparent with regard to current concepts of non-Hodgkin's lymphomas of childhood. These tumors, until only recently, were an ill-defined group of malignant neoplasms typically hidden within classifications of adult lymphomas. We now recognize two entities that represent the majority of childhood non-Hodgkin's lymphomas, namely, Burkitt's lymphoma[3] and lymphoblastic lymphoma.[4] These should be included in modern classifications of the non-Hodgkin's lymphomas as morphologically and clinically distinct neoplasms.

It has been our experience that the classification originally proposed by Rappaport,[5] with the modifications suggested by Dorfman,[6] not only can be readily employed by pathologists, but also appears to be relevant clinically. The classification we have found to be useful, and which can be consistently applied, is presented in Table 1. While the Rappaport classification is widely used, the terminology is clearly dated by relying solely on morphologic criteria.

TABLE 1
Classification of the Non-Hodgkin's Lymphomas

A. Nodular (follicular) lymphomas
   1. Lymphocytic, poorly differentiated
   2. Mixed lymphocytic–"histiocytic"
   3. "Histiocytic"

B. Diffuse lymphomas
   1. Lymphocytic, well-differentiated
   2. Lymphocytic, intermediate differentiation
   3. Lymphocytic, poorly differentiated
   4. Mixed lymphocytic–"histiocytic"
   5. "Histiocytic"
   6. Undifferentiated, Burkitt's type
   7. Undifferentiated, pleomorphic (non-Burkitt's)
   8. Lymphoblastic

C. Unclassified

It is now evident that the vast majority of so-called malignant lymphomas of "histiocytic" type are really comprised of neoplastic lymphocytes.[7] Furthermore, there is no strict scientific justification for the assessment of the degree of differentiation, that is, well, intermediately, poorly, and undifferentiated. These designations were based on morphologic observations of both normal and neoplastic lymphoid tissue. Whether a "well-differentiated" lymphocyte is more or less differentiated than an "undifferentiated" Burkitt's tumor cell or a "poorly differentiated lymphocyte" remains to be determined. Nevertheless, in spite of weaknesses in language, this modified classification appears to have clinical relevance and applicability within the framework of our present understanding of the pathobiology of non-Hodgkin's lymphomas.

The non-Hodgkin's lymphomas of childhood are distinct from those seen in adults. While approximately half of adult non-Hodgkin's lymphomas are nodular (follicular), this pattern is almost never observed in patients under the age of 15.[8] Among diffuse non-Hodgkin's lymphomas are the lymphocytic lymphomas (consisting of well, intermediately, and poorly differentiated forms) and mixed lymphocytic-"histiocytic" lymphomas. These tumors likewise are exceedingly unusual in children. The remaining four types of classifiable non-Hodgkin's lymphomas (Table 1) do occur during childhood and represent the vast majority of childhood non-Hodgkin's lymphomas. In western countries, approximately one-third of childhood non-Hodgkin's lymphomas are Burkitt's lymphomas, another one-third are lymphoblastic lymphomas, and the remaining are either undifferentiated pleomorphic (non-Burkitt's) or "histiocytic" lymphomas.[9] These neoplasms share several features in common that are not encountered in most adult non-Hodgkin's lymphomas. These special features include a diffuse growth pattern, a high growth fraction (high mitotic index), a propensity for extranodal involvement (30–50%) and early wide dissemination. Despite similarities, these lesions can be distinguished and separated into distinct entities by carefully applied morphologic criteria in association with immunologic and cytochemical observations.

UNDIFFERENTIATED LYMPHOMA, BURKITT'S TYPE

The entity now recognized as Burkitt's tumor first received close scrutiny in 1958 from Denis Burkitt, a British surgeon working in Uganda. He reported that "round cell" sarcomas occurred with extraordinary frequency in the jaws of children in tropical East Africa.[10] O'Conor and Davies subsequently reviewed all childhood tumors in the Uganda Cancer Registry and made the startling observation that fully 50% of them were malignant lymphomas of a rather uniform and "primitive" cell type.[11] The clinical presentations were remarkably stereotyped,[12] with facial and/or abdominal tumors predominating (Fig. 1). Facial tumors were especially characteristic of the youngest patients while abdominal tumors increased in frequency with age. In both surgical specimens and autopsies the tumors had distinctive gross and microscopic features.[13]

The distribution of patients within Africa, as well as the discovery of similar cases in New Guinea, suggested an intriguing geographical relationship between this lymphoma "syndrome" and conditions of temperature, altitude, and rainfall conducive to the propagation of endemic malaria. Epidemiologists suggested the possibility of an arthropod-borne vector as the causative agent of the disease. Excitement peaked in 1964, when Epstein, Achong, and Barr first observed in a cultured Burkitt's cell line the herpes-type virus now known as Epstein-Barr virus (EBV).[14]

There immediately arose the question whether this lymphoma was unique and restricted to certain "endemic" regions of the world or whether it could also be recognized and diagnosed elsewhere. The latter seemed to be the case when O'Conor[15] and Dorfman,[16] both fully familiar with the tumor in African patients, independently reported similar cases in retrospective reviews of childhood lymphomas in the United States. In the ensuing years there appeared a plethora of reports of "African lymphoma" or "Burkitt's tumor" from many countries, often proffered by authors who had never personally examined an African case. Great emphasis was placed on the clinical presentation with facial tumors, and yet it was known in Africa that patients clinically suspected of having Burkitt's tumor might prove histologically to have a variety of other entities (dentigerous cyst, ossifying fibroma, chloroma, retinoblastoma, embryonal rhabdomyosarcoma, a histologically different type of lymphoma, etc.). Confusion and controversy mounted, to the utter frustration of oncologists, epidemiologists, virologists, immunologists, and others committed to unraveling the mystery of "Burkitt's tumor."

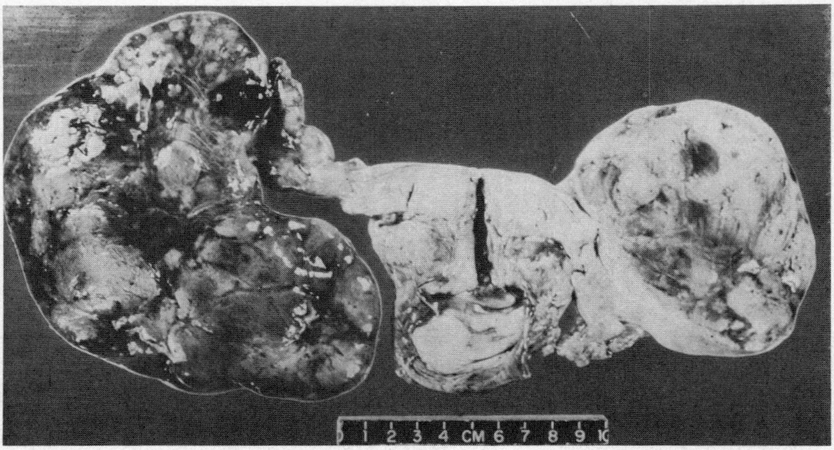

FIG. 1. Burkitt's lymphoma. Bilateral ovarian involvement in an American girl.

Scientists turned to the World Health Organization (WHO) for help in determining whether this tumor was a clinical syndrome, a clinicopathological syndrome, or a pathological entity. An expert committee commissioned by the WHO conducted a detailed and objective study of cases gathered from Africa and other countries and met in 1967 to formalize their conclusions. It was the consensus of the committee that Burkitt's tumor is a recognizable pathological entity,[3] with cytologic features distinct from those of other poorly differentiated lymphomas and leukemias. On morphological grounds alone, the cells could not be clearly assigned to any known pathway of differentiation, and it was recommended that the tumor be referred to as "malignant lymphoma, undifferentiated, Burkitt's type."[3]

The disease is usually characterized by rapidly growing solid tumors, with a normal or a leukoerythroblastic blood picture, which is secondary to marrow involvement by tumor. However, a small percentage of such patients, about 5%, eventually manifest neoplastic cells in the peripheral blood, usually as a terminal phase of disseminated visceral disease. A frankly leukemic presentation is distinctly rare. Thus in a large series of patients with acute nonmyelogenous leukemia, only 2% had blasts with the immunologic and cytologic features of Burkitt's tumor cells.[17]

Histologically, Burkitt's tumors from all parts of the world are indistinguishable. They are characteristically diffuse, with a monotonous proliferation of neoplastic cells and interspersed "starry sky" macrophages (Fig. 2 and Table 2).

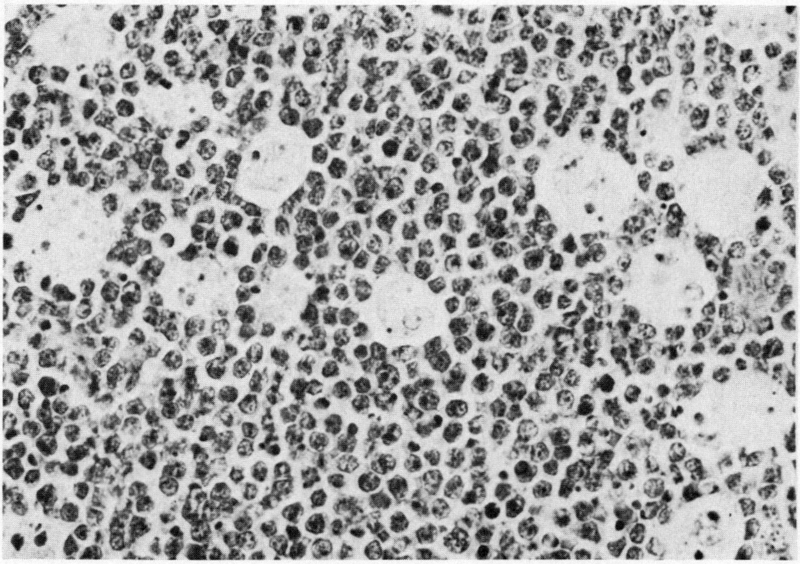

FIG. 2. Burkitt's lymphoma. Typical "starry-sky" pattern at low magnification. The clear zones contain benign macrophages with phagocytosed cellular fragments. (H&E, reduced from ×350)

The high growth fraction of Burkitt's tumor is manifested in the high mitotic index (approximately 4% of neoplastic cells) and the associated macrophages, which contain phagocytosed nuclear debris. The nuclei are round or oval and approximate the nuclear size of the "starry sky" macrophages (Fig. 3). Within the nuclei are two to five basophilic nucleoli and coarsely reticulated chromatin (Fig. 4). The distinct rim of amphophilic cytoplasm contains abundant RNA (Fig. 5) in the form of monoribosomes and polyribosomes (Fig. 6). Clear cytoplasmic vacuoles,

TABLE 2

Comparison of Morphology, Immunotype, and Cytochemistry of Childhood non-Hodgkin's Lymphomas[a]

Types of lymphomas	Histologic location when involvement is focal	Mitoses and starry sky	Nuclear size relative to macrophage nucleus	Chromatin	Nucleoli	Cytoplasm	Immunotype	MGP	TdT	AP
Burkitt's lymphoma	B-cell area (germinal centers)		Approximately same in all cells	Coarsely reticulated	+ (2–5)	Distinct but not abundant	B	++	–	–
Lympho-blastic lymphoma	T-cell area (paracortex)	+	Median smaller but variable from cell to cell	Finely dispersed	Incon-spicuous	Scant	T	±	+	+
Undiffer-entiated non-Burkitt's lymphoma	Variable	+	Median approx-imately same but variable cell to cell	Reticulated to vesicular	±	May be abundant	B or null	±/++	–	–
Histiocytic lymphoma	Variable; may be solitary	±	Median larger but variable from cell to cell	Reticulated to vesicular	+	May be abundant	B most often; null com-monly; T occasionally; histiocytic rarely	±/++		-/++

[a]Abbreviations: MGP = methyl green pyronin; TdT = terminal deoxynucleotidyl transferase; AP = acid phosphatase.

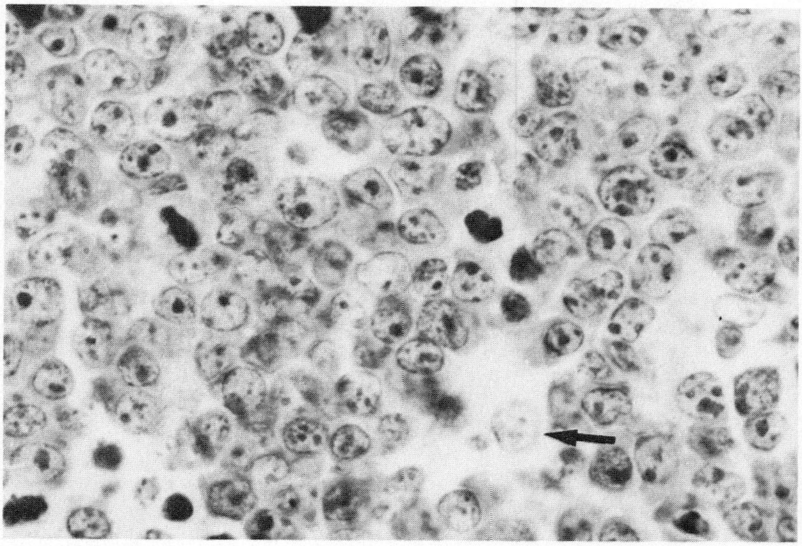

FIG. 3. Burkitt's lymphoma. The neoplastic cells are of relatively uniform size and shape. The diameters of the nuclei are in the same size range as those of the interspersed macrophages (arrow). Several small nucleoli and clumped chromatin are characteristic features of Burkitt's lymphoma cells. Numerous mitotic figures are present in this field. (H&E, reduced from ×950)

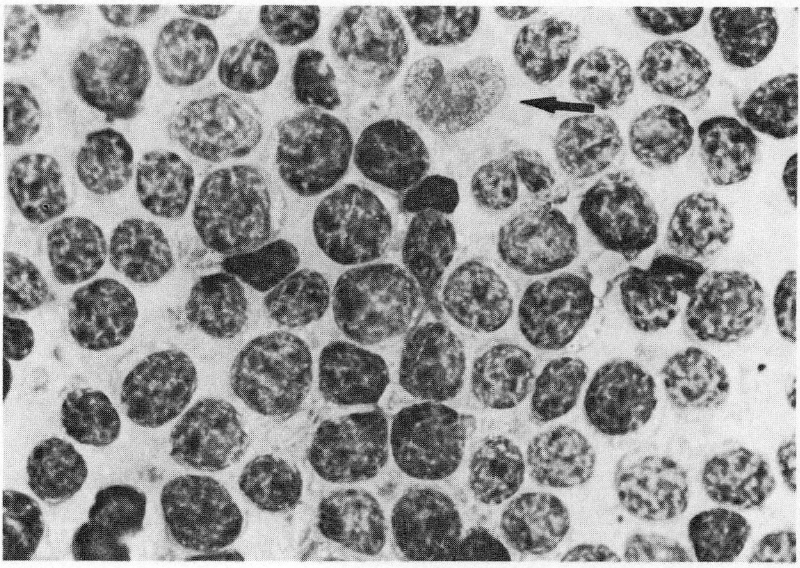

FIG. 4. Burkitt's lymphoma. The coarse chromatin and multiple nucleoli of Burkitt's lymphoma cells are readily appreciated in an imprint preparation. Cytoplasmic vacuoles may be present. A macrophage (arrow) provides comparison of nuclear size. (Wright's stain, reduced from ×950)

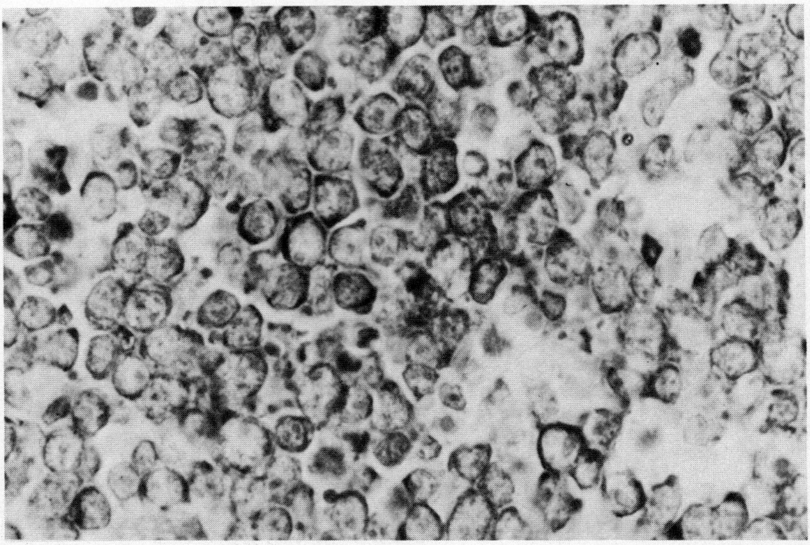

FIG. 5. Burkitt's lymphoma. Burkitt's lymphoma cells exhibit intense pyroninophilia in tissue sections such as this, as well as in imprints. The cytoplasm is uniformly and deeply stained and a distinct ring circumscribes the nucleus. (Methyl green pyronin stain, reduced from ×950)

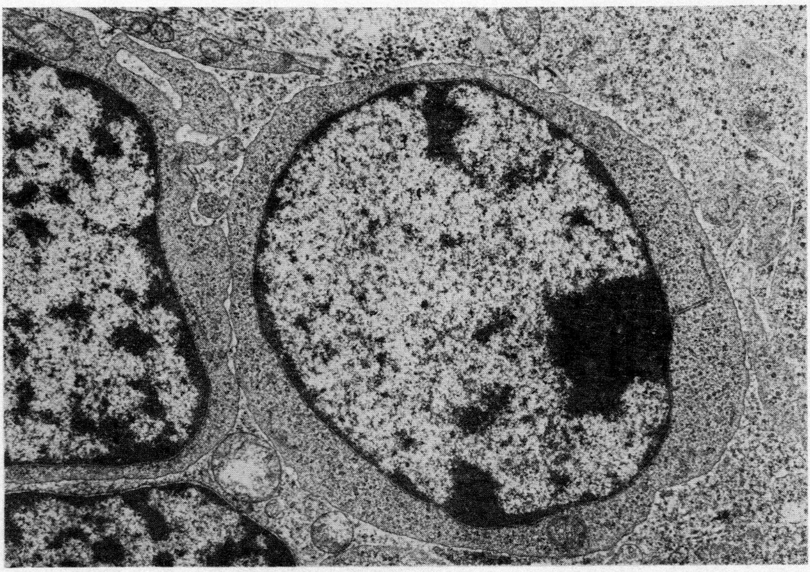

FIG. 6. Burkitt's lymphoma. Ultrastructurally, Burkitt's cells are characterized by multiple small nucleoli and clumped chromatin. The cytoplasm is rich in free ribosomes. Occasional strands of rough endoplasmic reticulum are present. (Uranyl acetate, lead citrate preparation, reduced from ×10,000. Courtesy of Dr. A. Julian Garvin, Laboratory of Pathology, NCI, NIH)

sometimes seen in paraffin sections, are often present in air-dried imprints. Many of these vacuoles contain neutral lipid; however, identical vacuoles can be observed in the neoplastic cells of other non-Hodgkin's lymphomas. Typically, the cytoplasm contains scant hydrolytic enzyme activity and no glycogen.

The B-cell nature of both endemic and nonendemic Burkitt's tumor has been clearly established.[17-20] Surface immunoglobulin (sIg) is readily demonstrated on the neoplastic cells and is usually restricted to a single light and heavy chain class (most commonly mu-kappa) within a given case. In addition, a variable percentage of the malignant cells possess receptors for the Fc fragment of IgG and for complement components C3b and/or C3d,[20,21] which are findings further indicative of their B-lymphocytic lineage.[20] Although Burkitt's tumor nearly always manifests a diffuse growth pattern, evidence is accumulating that it may be composed of cells derived from germinal centers. As initially pointed out by Lukes and Collins, the neoplastic cells resemble some small noncleaved cells observed in reactive germinal centers.[22] In a combined immunologic and morphologic study, Mann *et al*. were able to detect selective involvement of germinal centers in 10 out of 47 biopsy specimens and in 2 out of 17 autopsy specimens (Fig. 7).[20] It could not be determined whether the tumor cells were arising from or homing to these sites, but it is quite clear that the neoplastic cells are in some way related to B lymphocytes of normal germinal centers. Further support for this concept has been provided by the observation of Catovsky *et al*. of a follicular lymphoma that transformed to a lymphoma morphologically typical of Burkitt's tumor.[23]

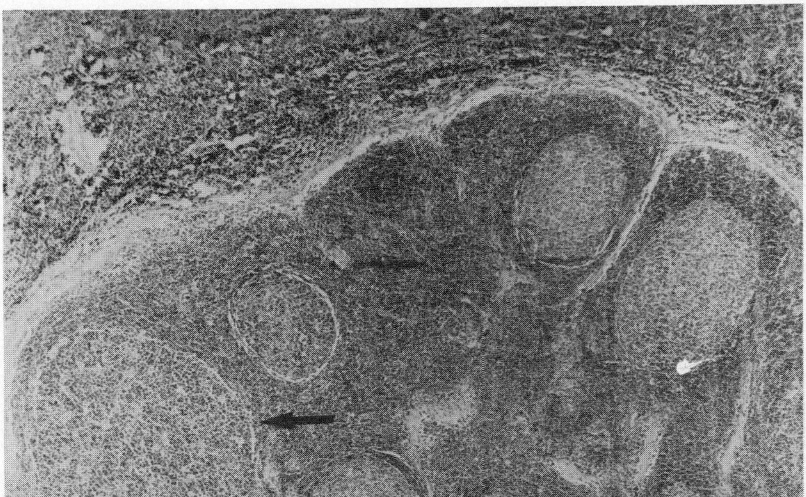

FIG. 7. Burkitt's lymphoma. Partial involvement of a mesenteric lymph node by Burkitt's lymphoma. A germinal center is selectively involved by lymphoma (arrow) and a monotonous, "starry-sky" pattern is evident at low magnification. The remainder of the lymph node contains germinal centers that are "polarized," i.e., the density of the cell population is greater toward the center of the lymph node. Such polarization is not present in the area involved by Burkitt's lymphoma. (H&E stain, reduced from ×40)

LYMPHOBLASTIC LYMPHOMA

The entity now recognized as lymphoblastic lymphoma has been referred to by a variety of terms, including Sternberg sarcoma, lymphosarcoma of childhood, convoluted lymphocytic lymphoma, and poorly differentiated lymphocytic lymphoma of childhood. The distinctive clinical, histologic, and immunologic characteristics of lymphoblastic lymphoma have resulted in the recent definition of this lymphoma as a clinicopathologic entity.[4] It most commonly occurs in adolescents and young adults, although it has been observed in the elderly as well.[4]

The common mode of presentation differs from Burkitt's tumor. Thus lymphoblastic lymphomas are characterized by supradiaphragmatic lymphadenopathy with involvement of cervical, axillary, and/or supraclavicular lymph nodes, and they often occur in association with an anterior mediastinal mass (50% of cases) and malignant pleural effusion. Rarely do they occur in the gastrointestinal tract. In addition, dissemination to bone marrow and peripheral blood with progression to acute lymphoblastic leukemia (ALL) is seen in as many as one-half of the cases.[24-26] The frequent occurrence of such a leukemic picture and the morphologic overlap between the blasts of acute lymphoblastic leukemia and the cells of lymphoblastic lymphoma have led observers to the conclusion that the two presentations are simply different initial manifestations of a single neoplastic disorder.[27-31] This situation is analogous to the relationship of chronic lymphocytic leukemia and diffuse well-differentiated lymphocytic lymphoma in adults.

Lymphoblastic lymphoma grows in a diffuse, monotonous pattern often with interspersed "starry-sky" macrophages. In contrast to Burkitt's lymphoma, partially involved lymph nodes demonstrate selective distribution of the neoplastic cells in paracortical T-cell areas (Fig. 8 and Table 2). Compared to Burkitt's lymphoma, the cytoplasm is scant; in addition, pyroninophilia is not as marked, and PAS positive, diastase-sensitive granules may be present, particularly in imprint preparations. The nuclei may vary in size and shape, and many cases exhibit markedly irregular nuclear contours or "convolutions" (Fig. 9–11). Although Lukes and his associates[30-32] have identified nuclear convolutions in nearly all cases of lymphoblastic lymphoma, in our experience and in that of others,[4] nuclear convolutions may not be evident in as many as half the cases (Fig. 12). There appears to be considerable variation, since both convoluted and nonconvoluted forms may be present in the same section, with smaller cells being the most markedly convoluted.[33] Whether or not the cells are convoluted, the patients are virtually indistinguishable in mode of presentation and in clinical behavior.[4] Thus we may be observing a spectrum of cytology within one disease entity, and the nuclear convolutions, when present, merely serve to confirm the diagnosis. The nuclear chromatin is characteristically fine and evenly dispersed and nucleoli are inconspicuous or absent, imparting a blastic appearance to the neoplastic cells (Fig. 9 and 10).

Most cases of lymphoblastic lymphoma are of T-cell origin,[7,28,29,31-34] as demonstrated by their ability to form spontaneous rosettes with sheep erythro-

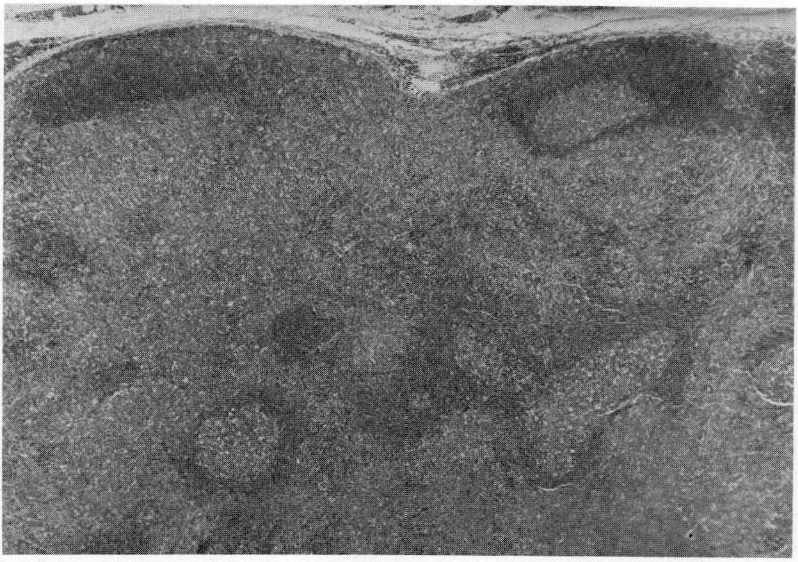

FIG. 8. Lymphoblastic lymphoma. This lymphoma exhibits a diffuse growth pattern, selective involvement of paracortical (T-cell) areas, and sparing of the outer cortex and germinal center (B-cell) areas. (H&E stain, reduced from ×40)

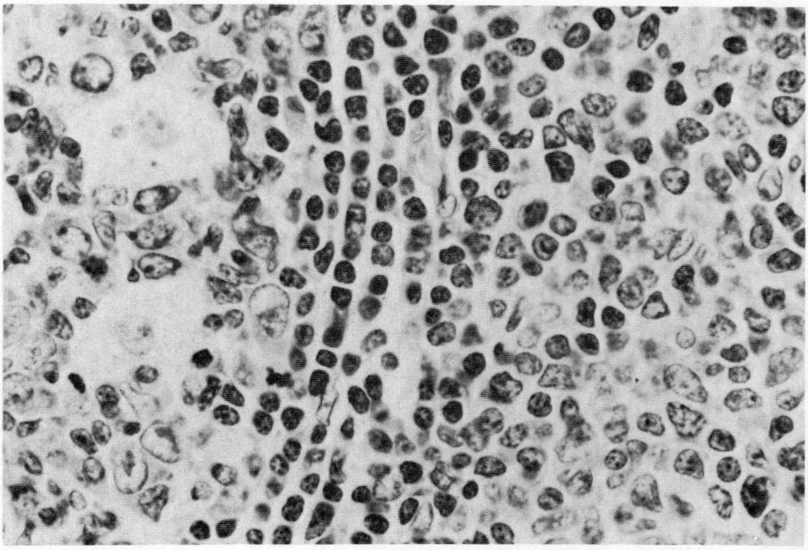

FIG. 9. Lymphoblastic lymphoma. Lymph node with partial involvement by lymphoblastic lymphoma (right), which is adjacent to a germinal center (left). The mature appearance of the small lymphocytes of the mantle zone contrasts with that of the nuclei of the neoplastic cells. (H&E stain, reduced from ×750)

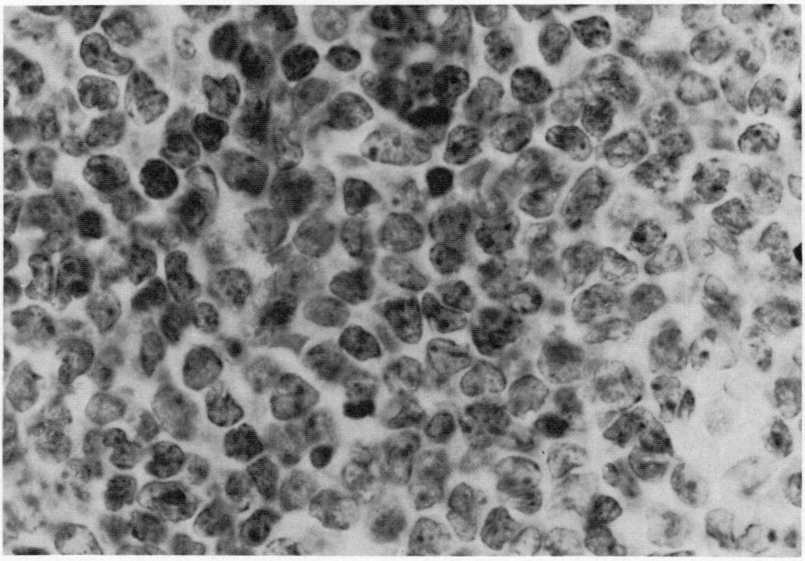

FIG. 10. Lymphoblastic lymphoma. Most cells have convoluted nuclei and small, inconspicuous nucleoli. (H&E stain, reduced from ×950)

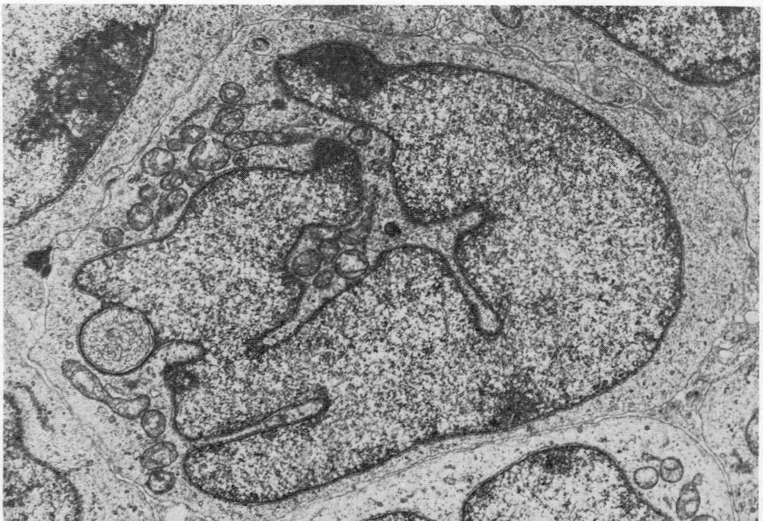

FIG. 11. Lymphoblastic lymphoma. This figure shows that complex nuclear convolutions in lymphoblastic lymphona are sometimes best appreciated by electron microscopy. Numerous mitochrondria and free ribosomes are present in the cytoplasm. Rough endoplasmic reticulum is usually scant or absent. (Uranyl acetate, lead citrate preparation, reduced from ×10,600. Courtesy of Dr. A. Julian Garvin, Laboratory of Pathology, NCI, NIH)

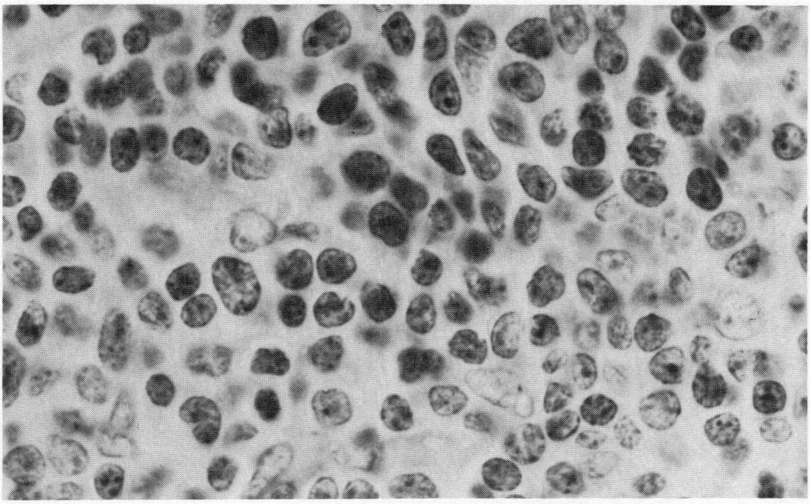

FIG. 12. Lymphoblastic lymphoma. Some cases are characterized by cells with round or oval (nonconvoluted) nuclear shapes and only occasional nuclear identations. The indistinct small nucleoli, evenly dispersed chromatin and scant cytoplasm distinguish this lesion from Burkitt's lymphoma. (H&E stain, reduced from ×950)

cytes (E rosettes) (Fig. 13A), by the presence of human T-lymphocyte-associated antigens (HTLA),[35] and by the absence of surface immunoglobulin.[28,29,33-36] These observations are not unexpected, since lymphoblastic lymphoma has a propensity for infiltration of T-dependent paracortical areas of lymph nodes and anterior mediastinal involvement.

The fact that both lymphoblastic lymphoma and T-cell ALL are of T-cell origin is further evidence that they are clinically different manifestations of a single disease entity. They share several features in common, such as a high male to female ratio, a tendency for occurrence in age groups older than typical for common (or null cell) ALL, white blood cell counts frequently greater than $100{,}000/mm^3$, and a poor prognosis with frequent early central nervous system involvement. Most cases also demonstrate nuclear terminal deoxynucleotidyl transferase (TdT)[36] (Fig. 13B), punctate cytoplasmic acid phosphatase (Fig. 13C) and beta-glucuronidase activity. Suppressor cell activity[37] has been described for T-cell ALL. Notably, the cells from many cases of both lymphoblastic lymphoma and T-cell ALL possess receptors for the C3 component of complement[7,29,34,38] (Fig. 14). This observation initially appeared paradoxical since C3 receptors are found on most normal peripheral B-lymphocytes and monocytes but not on T-lymphocytes.[39,40] However, complement receptors have subsequently been detected on rare normal T-lymphocytes from peripheral blood and lymphoid tissue (so-called "D" lymphocytes)[41] and on fetal thymocytes.[42,43] Thus T-cell ALL and lymphoblastic lymphoma both represent a neoplastic proliferation of primitive thymic dependent lymphocytes.

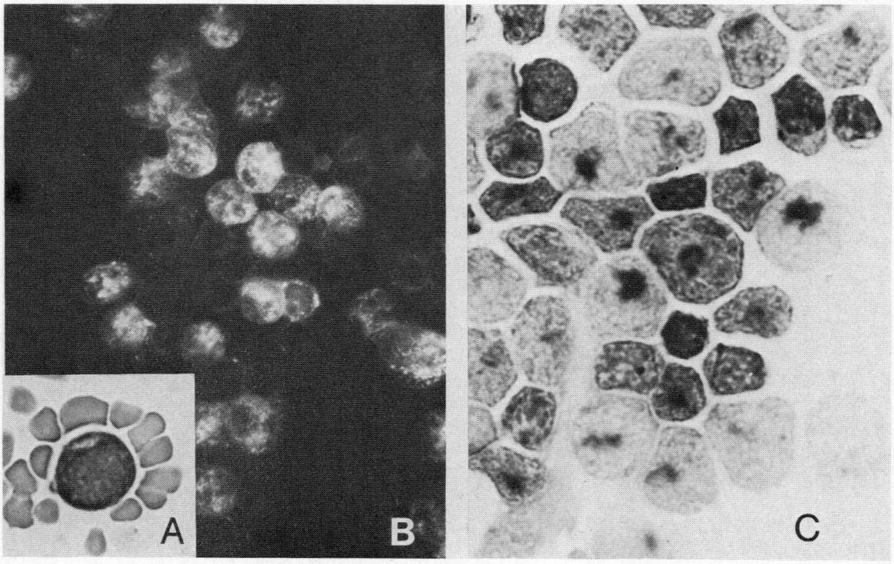

FIG. 13. Lymphoblastic lymphoma. (A) E-rosette formation in lymphoblastic lymphoma. Rosettes formed in suspension of viable cells are cytocentrifuged and stained with Wright's stain. This procedure permits confirmation that the rosetted cells are neoplastic and not normal T cells. (Wright's stain, reduced from ×950. Courtesy of Dr. Elaine S. Jaffe, Laboratory of Pathology, NCI, NIH) (B) Detection of intranuclear terminal deoxynucleotidyl transferase (TdT) by indirect immunofluorescence of a cytocentrifuge preparation of a cellular suspension of lymphoblastic lymphoma. A coarsely reticular pattern of staining is evident in the nuclei of the neoplastic cells. (UV epifluorescence stain, reduced from ×480. Courtesy of Dr. Fred Bollum, Uniformed Services University of the Health Sciences) (C) Intense, punctate juxtanuclear cytoplasmic staining for acid phosphatase; this is often observed in lymphoblastic lymphoma. (HPR stain, reduced from ×950. Courtesy of Dr. Thomas Callihan, Laboratory of Pathology, NCI, NIH)

Approximately one-third of the cases of lymphoblastic lymphoma are immunologically null, that is, devoid of cell surface markers.[32,33] These non-T, non-B cases are morphologically heterogeneous, i.e., nuclear convolutions are present in some cases but not in others.[32,33] The subjective interpretation of nuclear convolutions is reflected by contradictory findings in the literature. In an ultrastructural study, Glick *et al.* observed nuclear convolutions in ALL regardless of immunotype, but these authors indicated that "nuclear irregularity appeared most extreme within the non-T, non-B group."[33] Conversely, by light microscopy, Williams *et al.* detected T-cell markers on the neoplastic cells of five out of seven "convoluted lymphoma/leukemia" cases, but three out of these five cases had 10% or fewer E rosettes. Furthermore, 7 out of 36 "nonconvoluted" cases had T-cell markers.[32]

Thus we believe it is too early to make definite statements correlating surface markers with morphology for lymphoblastic lymphoma and ALL. The position of the non-T, non-B subtype within lymphoblastic lymphoma will undoubtedly be

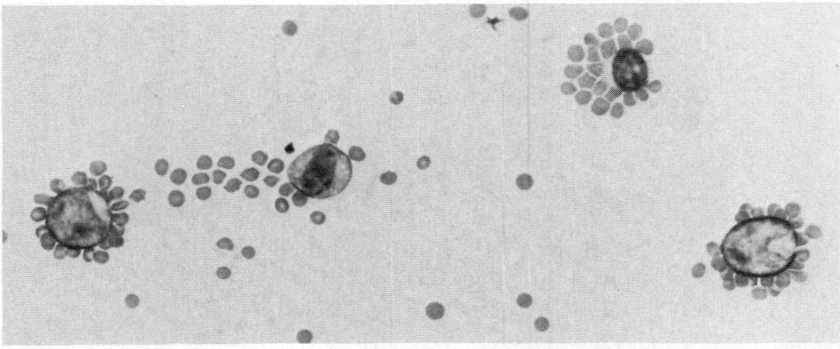

FIG. 14. Lymphoblastic lymphoma. This figure shows neoplastic cells forming rosettes with EAC (sheep erythrocytes coated with IgM antibody and complement), indicating surface receptors for complement. (Wright's stain, reduced from ×650)

clarified by further investigation. At present the designation "unclassified" lymphoblastic lymphoma may be preferable to "null" cell, to avoid confusing these tumors with null cell (common) ALL. The evidence to date has not demonstrated clinical differences between T-cell lymphoblastic lymphoma and non-T, non-B (unclassified) lymphoblastic lymphoma. Therefore, an analogy should not be drawn between these lesions and T-cell *versus* common (null cell) ALL, in which the T-cell ALL cases have a poorer prognosis.[44,45] The survival difference between these two types of ALL correlates with the initial white blood cell count, which is probably the single most significant prognostic factor for ALL.[44]

LARGE CELL ("HISTIOCYTIC") AND UNDIFFERENTIATED, PLEOMORPHIC (NON-BURKITT'S) LYMPHOMAS

The so-called "histiocytic" and undifferentiated pleomorphic (non-Burkitt's) lymphomas represent approximately one-third of childhood non-Hodgkin's lymphomas. They are a morphologically heterogeneous group of tumors, and the cytologic polymorphism of the undifferentiated non-Burkitt's and the large cell ("histiocytic") lymphomas is mirrored in their clinical and immunologic diversity. Unlike the lymphoblastic and Burkitt's groups, these tumors have not been associated with characteristic clinical features. They appear in all stages in a broad spectrum of sites, including the nasopharynx, tonsils, gastrointestinal tract, lung, mediastinum, bone, gonads, skin, and soft tissue. Although clinically aggressive, they have been encouragingly responsive to modern intensive combination chemotherapy.[46,47] There is considerable morphologic overlap between these two, and the distinction relies mainly on cellular size. Both are seen more commonly in adults, in contrast to Burkitt's lymphoma and lymphoblastic lymphoma. Unlike nodular lymphomas, these tumors tend to involve extranodal sites and grow as large circumscribed masses when invading the spleen and other organs (Fig. 15).

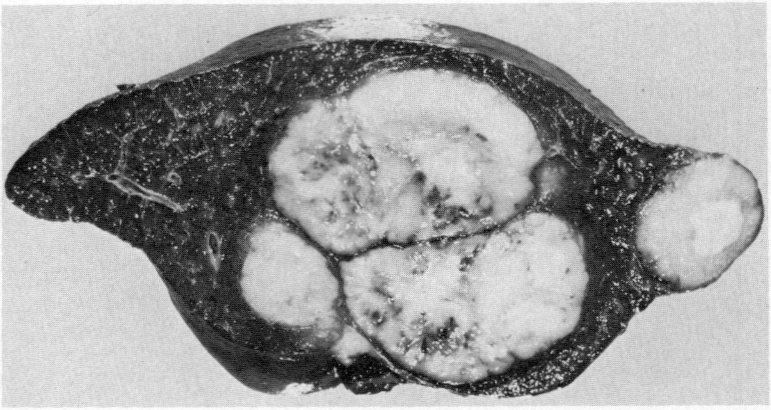

FIG. 15. Large cell (''histiocytic'') lymphoma. Large tumorous masses in the spleen.

The ''histiocytic'' lymphomas are morphologically diverse, but the vast majority are lymphoid in origin.[7,48] Thus we prefer the term ''large lymphoid'' as proposed by Dorfman[6] rather than the misnomers ''histiocytic'' lymphoma and ''reticulum cell'' sarcoma. The nuclei are vesicular, with one to three nucleoli often apposed to the inner surface of the nuclear membrane (Fig. 16). These large nuclei may manifest clefts (Fig. 17), which are an essential feature of the large

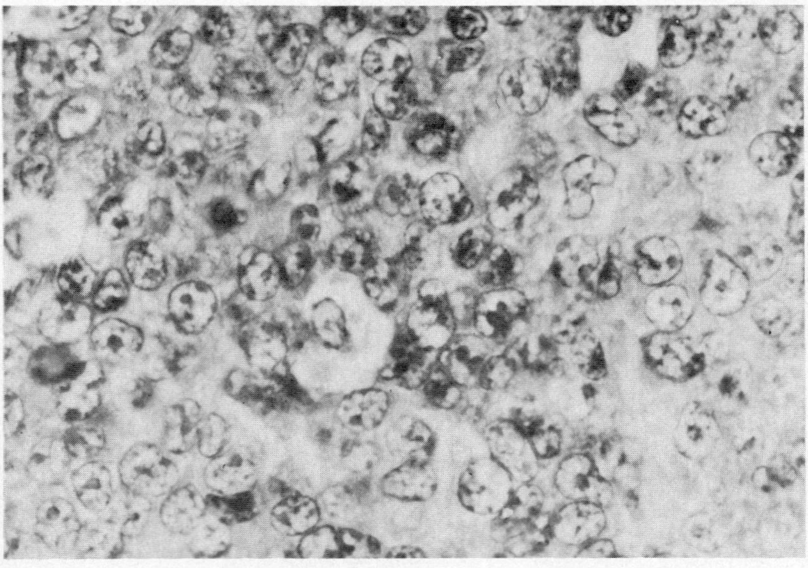

FIG. 16. Large cell (''histiocytic'') lymphoma. The nuclei are often round (noncleaved) and vesicular, and contain readily detectable nucleoli. (H&E stain, reduced from ×950)

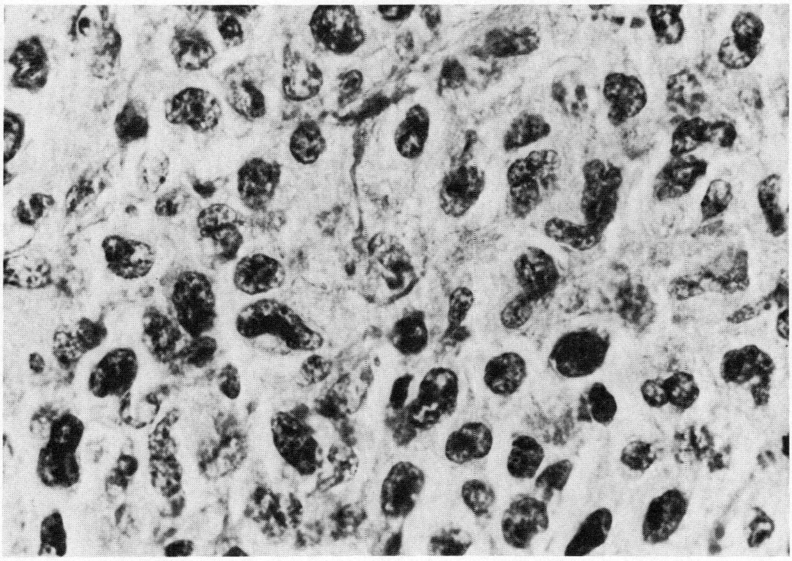

FIG. 17. Large cell (''histiocytic'') lymphoma. Large cleaved cells predominate. (H&E stain, reduced from ×950)

cleaved follicular center cells of Lukes.[49] But more often the large nuclei are noncleaved (Fig. 16). Although individual nuclear size is quite variable, the median is always greater than the diameter of the nuclei of accompanying benign macrophages, which are a common feature of these lesions. Mitotic figures are numerous and multinuclear forms may occur. The cytoplasm is abundant and ranges from clear to amphophilic, imparting a ''histiocytic'' appearance to the neoplastic cells.

Undifferentiated non-Burkitt's lymphomas (UDNB) superficially resemble Burkitt's lymphomas, and these two can be rather difficult to distinguish at times. However, undifferentiated non-Burkitt's lymphomas occur at all ages while Burkitt's tumor is rare over the age of 30 (Table 3).[50] In addition, UDNB regardless of age exhibits a poorer long-term survival than Burkitt's lymphomas (Fig. 18).[50] At low magnification the presence of a ''starry-sky'' pattern reminiscent of Burkitt's lymphoma may be striking (Fig. 19). The median nuclear size is in the range of the neighboring macrophages and smaller than the nuclei of ''histiocytic'' lymphoma (Fig. 20A–C). However, unlike Burkitt's lymphoma, there is not a monotony of neoplastic cells but rather a considerable range of size and shape. In addition, binucleated and trinucleated cells may be present, and cytoplasm may be more abundant than in Burkitt's lymphoma. Since some cases of ''histiocytic'' lymphoma exhibit many of these features, the distinction between such tumors and undifferentiated non-Burkitt's lymphomas is made on the basis of nuclear size. Whether such a distinction is of clinical significance remains to be determined.

TABLE 3
Age Distribution of Undifferentiated Lymphomas at the National Cancer Institute

Types of lymphomas	Percent of cases by age (years)							
	<10	10–19	20–29	30–39	40–49	50–59	60–69	>70
Burkitt's Lymphoma (*n*=39, median= 8 years)	49	36	13	2	—	—	—	—
Undifferentiated non-Burkitt's lymphoma (*n*=27, median= 34 years)	11	19	15	11	11	7	15	11

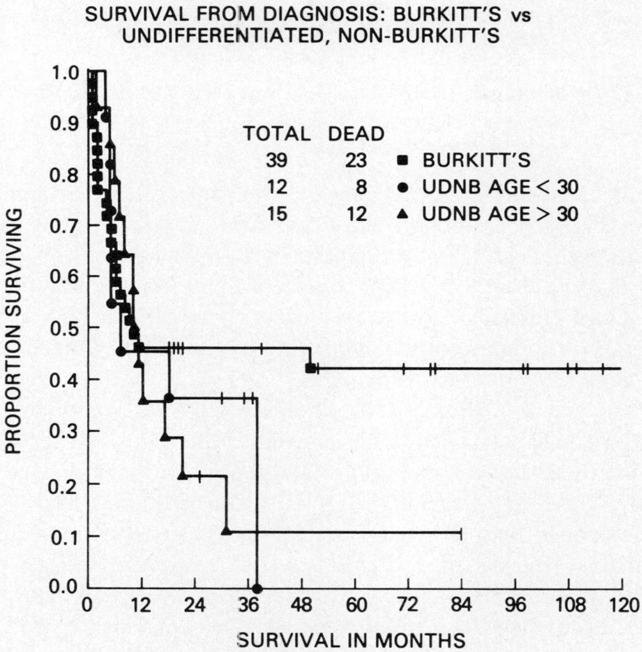

FIG. 18. Survival curves for Burkitt's lymphoma and undifferentiated non-Burkitt's lymphomas (UDNB). The undifferentiated non-Burkitt's patients have been divided into two groups by age. Patients with undifferentiated non-Burkitt's lymphoma, regardless of age, exhibit a poorer survival than those with Burkitt's lymphoma. Patients with Burkitt's lymphoma surviving for the first two years from diagnosis usually experienced prolonged survival. Solid symbols represent deaths and vertical marks represent the most recent point of follow-up. (Courtesy of Dr. A. Julian Garvin, Laboratory of Pathology, NCI, NIH)

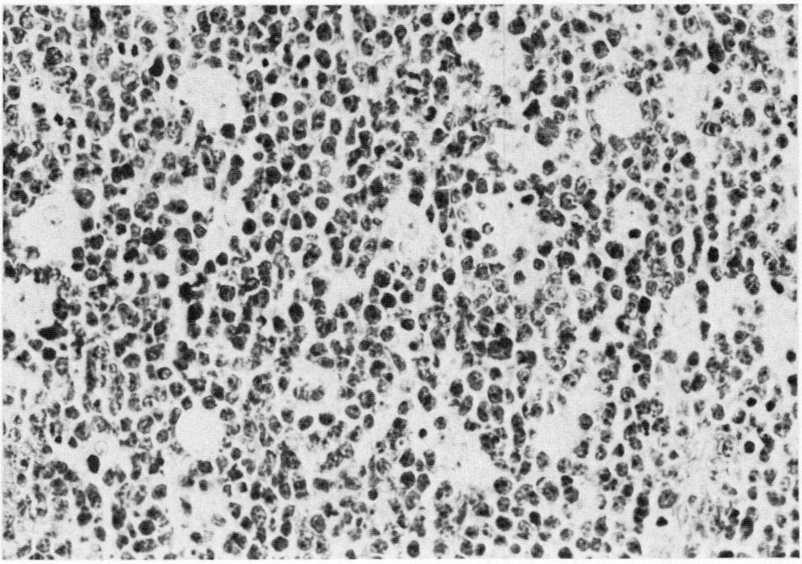

FIG. 19. Undifferentiated, non-Burkitt's lymphoma. Diffuse growth pattern with interspersed ''starry-sky'' macrophages in UDNB superficially resembles Burkitt's lymphoma. (H&E stain, reduced from ×100)

Most (50–60%) ''histiocytic'' lymphomas and undifferentiated non-Burkitt's lymphomas are of B-cell origin[48] and, in fact, it is not unusual to observe plasmacytoid features in the neoplastic cells of ''histiocytic'' lymphomas, particularly in adults. Immunoperoxidase staining of formalin fixed, paraffin-embedded tissue sections has revealed monoclonal intracytoplasmic immunoglobulin (cIg) in the neoplastic cells from numerous cases, even those lacking plasmacytoid features.[51-53] Such cells are presumably the neoplastic counterparts of B-immunoblasts that have begun to synthesize cIg in an abortive attempt toward plasma cell differentiation.

T-cell markers have been detected in 5–15% of the cases studied thus far.[48] True histiocytic large cell lymphomas have been rare.[54] One case of a lymphoma of true histiocytic origin occurred in the clavicle of a 14-year-old boy. The cells were large and contained abundant deeply eosinophilic cytoplasm (Fig. 21). The neoplastic cells not only formed rosettes with IgG-sensitized sheep erythrocytes and complement-coated sheep erythrocytes, but they also lacked surface immunoglobulin (sIg) and phagocytosed the sensitized red cells, further indications of their monocyte-macrophage origin (Fig. 21, inset). Cytoplasmic enzymes characteristic of monocytes and macrophages were also detected.

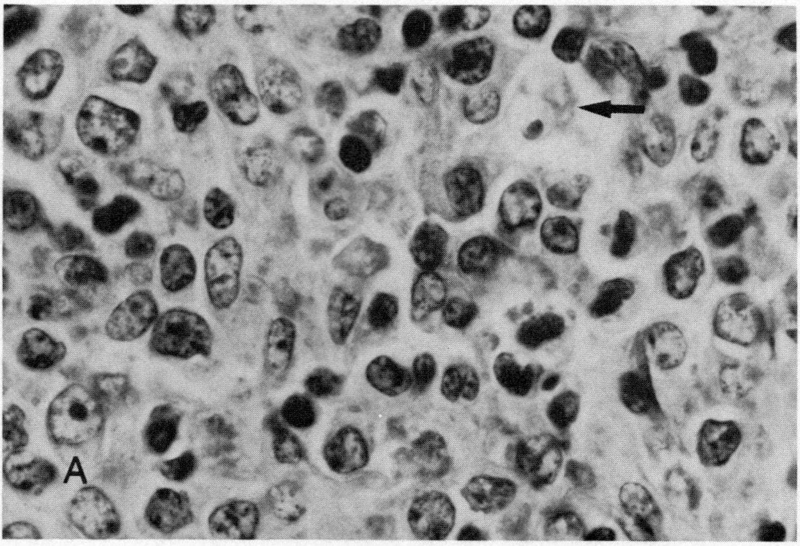

FIG. 20A.

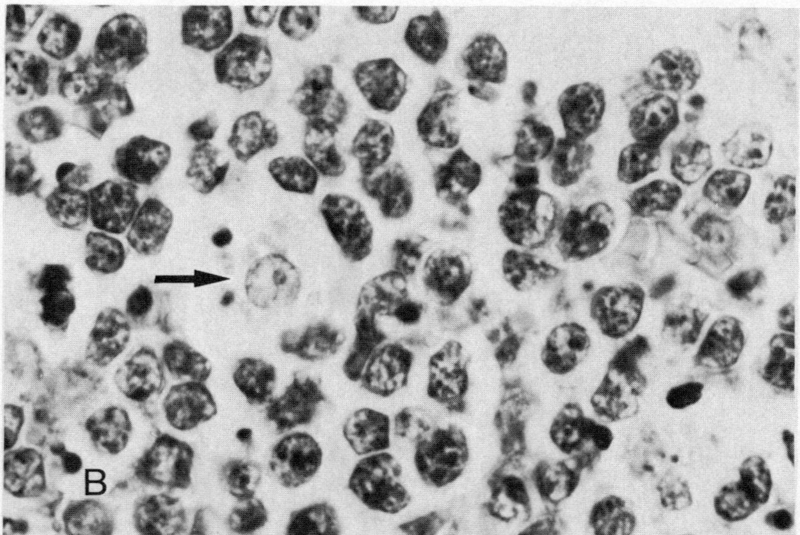

FIG. 20B.

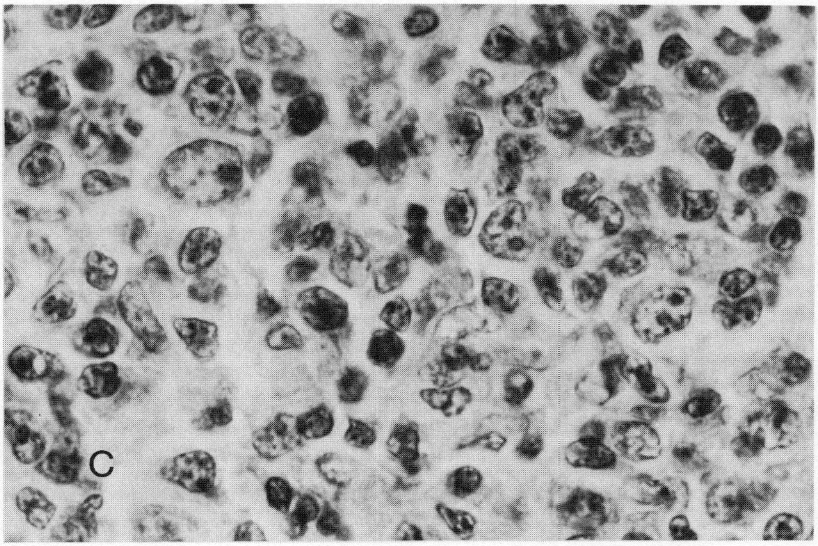

FIG. 20. Undifferentiated, non-Burkitt's lymphoma. Three different cases of UDNB demonstrate that this is not a morphologically homogeneous disorder. Nuclei vary in size and shape and may be rather irregular. The nuclear size range approximates that of macrophage nuclei (arrows in A and B). Prominent, single central nucleoli, which are not a feature of Burkitt's lymphoma, may be observed in UDNB. (H&E stain, all reduced from ×950)

SUMMARY

Non-Hodgkin's lymphomas are subdivided morphologically into two growth patterns, nodular and diffuse. The vast majority of childhood non-Hodgkin's lymphomas exhibit a diffuse growth pattern, often in association with a high growth fraction (high mitotic index) and a tendency for extranodal involvement. Approximately one-third of childhood non-Hodgkin's lymphomas in western countries are undifferentiated lymphomas of Burkitt's type and another one-third are lymphoblastic lymphomas. The remainder are largely comprised of undifferentiated pleomorphic (non-Burkitt's) lymphoma and large cell (''histiocytic'') lymphoma.

Our ability to classify the non-Hodgkin's lymphomas has been enhanced by recent advances in the immunologic identification of lymphoreticular cells. Newer immunological techniques, when applied to malignant lymphomas, have clearly established these tumors as neoplasms of the immune system. An integral approach, drawing upon morphological, functional and immunological features, offers new insights into the pathobiology of non-Hodgkin's lymphomas.

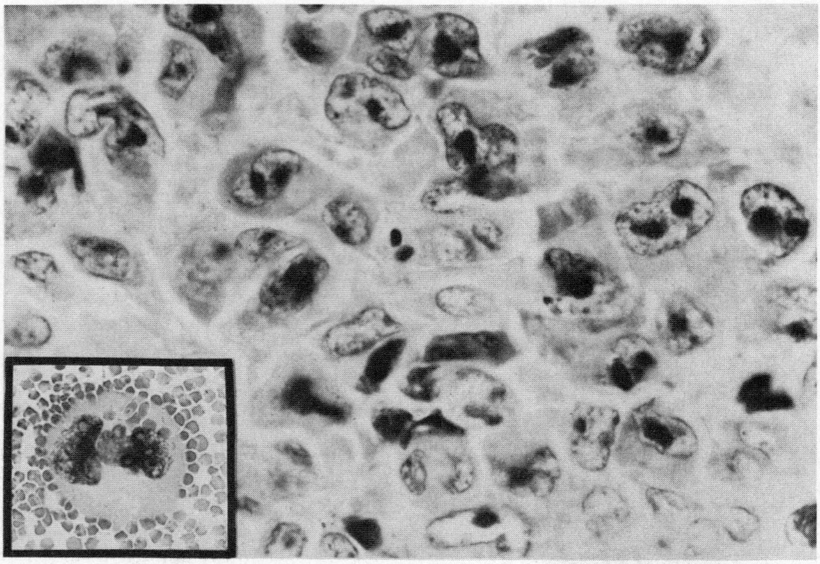

FIG. 21. Malignant lymphoma with true histiocytic markers. The neoplastic cells are large and pleomorphic with abundant cytoplasm and irregularly shaped nuclei. Neoplastic cells not only form rosettes with EAC but also phagocytize the complement-coated erythrocytes (inset). Such avid phagocytic activity is indicative of a cell of macrophage or histiocytic origin. (H&E stain, reduced from ×950; inset, Wright's stain, reduced from ×750. Inset courtesy of Dr. Elaine S. Jaffe, Laboratory of Pathology, NCI, NIH)

ACKNOWLEDGMENTS

The authors wish to thank Mr. Ralph Isenburg, who provided photographic assistance, and Mrs. Louise Longnecker, who typed the manuscript.

References

1. Cutler SJ, Young JL (eds): Third National Cancer Survey: Incidence Data. *Natl Cancer Inst Monogr 41:100–101, 1975.*
2. Sutow WW, Vietti TJ, Fernbach DJ (eds): *Clinical Pediatric Oncology.* C V Mosby, St. Louis, 1975, p. 2–3.
3. Berard CW, O'Conor GT, Thomas LB, *et al* (eds): Histopathological definition of Burkitt's tumour. *Bull WHO 40:601–607, 1969.*
4. Nathwani BN, Kim H, Rappaport H: Malignant lymphoma lymphoblastic. *Cancer 38:964–983, 1976.*
5. Rappaport H: *Tumors of the Hematopoietic System.* Atlas of Tumor Pathology, Section 3, Fascicle 8, Armed Forces Institute of Pathology, Washington, D.C., 1966.

6. Dorfman RF: Classification of non-Hodgkin's lymphomas. *Lancet 2:961–962, 1974.*
7. Jaffe ES, Braylan RC, Nanba K, *et al.*: Functional markers a new perspective on malignant lymphomas. *Cancer Treat Rep 61:953–962, 1977.*
8. Frizerra G, Murphy SB: Follicular (nodular) lymphoma in childhood, a rare clinical-pathological entity; report of eight cases from four cancer centers. *Cancer 44:2218–2235, 1979.*
9. Jaffe ES, Berard CW: Lymphoblastic lymphoma, a term rekindled with new precision. *Ann Intern Med 89:415–417, 1978.*
10. Burkitt D: A sarcoma involving the jaws in African children. *Br J Surg 46:218–223, 1958.*
11. O'Conor GT, Davies JNP: Malignant tumors in African children. *J. Pediatr 56:526, 1960.*
12. Burkitt D, O'Conor GT: Malignant lymphoma in African children. I. A clinical syndrome. *Cancer 14:258–269, 1961.*
13. O'Conor GT: Malignant lymphoma in African children. II. A pathological entity. *Cancer 14:270–283, 1961.*
14. Epstein MA, Achong BG, Barr YM: Virus-particles in cultured lymphoblasts from Burkitt's lymphoma. *Lancet 1:702–703, 1964.*
15. O'Conor GT, Rappaport H, Smith EB: Childhood lymphoma resembling "Burkitt tumor" in the United States. *Cancer 18:411–417, 1965.*
16. Dorfman RF: Childhood lymphosarcoma in St. Louis, Missouri, clinically and histologically resembling Burkitt's tumor. *Cancer 18:418–430, 1965.*
17. Flandrin G, Brouet JC, Daniel MT, *et al*: Acute leukemia with Burkitt's tumor cells; a study of six cases with special reference to lymphocyte surface markers. *Blood 45:183–188, 1975.*
18. Fialkow RJ, Klein E, Klein G, *et al*: Immunoglobulin and glucose-6-phosphate dehydrogenase as markers of cellular origin in Burkitt lymphoma. *J Exp Med 138:89–102, 1973.*
19. Binder RA, Jencks JA, Chun B, *et al*: "B" cell origin of malignant cells in a case of American Burkitt's lymphoma. *Cancer 36:161–168, 1975.*
20. Mann RB, Jaffe ES, Braylan RC, *et al*: Non-endemic Burkitt's lymphoma; a B-cell tumor related to germinal centers. *N Engl J Med 295:685–691, 1976.*
21. Shevach EM, Herberman R, Frank MM, *et al*: Receptors for complement and immunoglobulin on human leukemic cells and human lymphoblastoid cell lines. *J Clin Invest 51:1933–1938, 1972.*
22. Lukes RJ, Collins RD: New approaches to the classification of the lymphomata. *Br J Cancer 31(suppl. II):1–28, 1975.*
23. Catovsky D, Pittman S, Lewis E, *et al*: Marker chromosome 14q+ in follicular lymphoma in transformation. *Lancet 2:934, 1977.*
24. Webster R: Lymphosarcoma of the thymus; its relation to acute lymphatic leukemia. *Med J Aust 48:582–586, 1961.*
25. Davis LA, McCreadle SR: The enlarged thymus gland in leukemia in childhood. *Am J Roentgenol 88:924–927, 1962.*
26. Sullivan MP: Leukemic transformation in lymphosarcoma of childhood. *Pediatrics 29:589–599, 1962.*
27. Berard CW: Histopathology of the lymphomas, in Williams WJ Beutler E, Erslev AJ, *et al* (eds): *Hematology*. McGraw-Hill, New York, 1972, pp. 901–912.
28. Kaplan J, Mastrangelo R, Peterson WD Jr: Childhood lymphoblastic lymphoma, a cancer of thymus derived lymphocytes. *Cancer Res 34:521–525, 1974.*
29. Kersey J, Sabod A, Gajl-Peczalska KJ: Neoplastic cells from childhood lymphoblastic leukemia and lymphoma with T and B lymphocyte markers (abstract). *Am J Pathol 74:64, 1974.*
30. Barcos MP, Lukes RJ: Malignant lymphoma of convoluted lymphocytes: A new entity of possible T-cell type, in Sinks LF, Godden JO (eds): *Conflicts in Childhood Cancer: An Evaluation of Current Management*. Alan R Liss, New York, 1975, pp. 147–178.
31. Rosen PJ, Feinstein DI, Pattengale PK, *et al*: Convoluted lymphocytic lymphoma in adults; a clinicopathologic entity. *Ann Intern Med 89:319–324, 1978.*
32. Williams AH, Taylor CR, Higgins GR, *et al*: Childhood lymphoma-leukemia. I. Correlation of morphology and immunologic studies. *Cancer 42:171–181, 1978.*

33. Glick AD, Vestal BK, Flexner JM, *et al*: Ultrastructural study of acute lymphocytic leukemia; comparison with immunologic studies. *Blood 52:311–322, 1978.*
34. Jaffe ES, Braylan RC, Frank MM, *et al*: Heterogeneity of immunologic markers and surface morphology in childhood lymphoblastic lymphoma. *Blood 48:213–222, 1976.*
35. Kersey JH, Nesbit ME, Hallgren H, *et al*: Evidence for origin of certain childhood acute lymphoblastic leukemias and lymphomas from thymus derived lymphocytes. *Cancer 36:1348–1352, 1975.*
36. Donlon JA, Jaffe ES, Braylan RC: Terminal deoxynucleotidyl transferase activity in malignant lymphomas. *N Engl J Med 297:461–464, 1977.*
37. Broder S, Poplack D, Whang-Pheng J, *et al*: Characterization of a suppressor-cell leukemia; evidence for the requirement of an interaction of two T cells in development of human suppressor effector cells. *N Engl J Med 298:66–72, 1978.*
38. Cossman J, Schnitzer B, Deegan MJ: Immunologic surface markers in non-Hodgkin's lymphomas. *Am J Pathol 87:19–32, 1977.*
39. Nussenzweig V: Receptor for immune complexes on lymphocytes. *Adv Immunol 19:217–258, 1974.*
40. Ross GD, Rabellino EM, Polley MJ, *et al*: Combined studies of complement receptor and surface immunoglobulin-bearing cells and sheep erythrocyte rosette-forming cells in normal and leukemic human lymphocytes. *J Clin Invest 52:377–385, 1973.*
41. Barret SG: Tissue distribution of human T cells with complement receptors (D cells). *Clin Immunol Immunopathol 11:190–195, 1978.*
42. Gatien JG, Schneeberger EE, Parkman R, *et al*: Isolation on discontinuous gradients of bovine albumin of a subpopulation of human lymphocytes exhibiting precursor characteristics. *Eur J Immunol 5:306–312, 1977.*
43. Stein H, Muller-Hermelink HK: Simultaneous presence of receptors for complement and sheep red blood cells on human fetal thymocytes. *Br J Haematol 36:225–230, 1977.*
44. Chessells JM, Hardisty RM, Rapson NT, *et al*: Acute lymphoblastic leukemia in children; classification and prognosis. *Lancet 2:1307–1309, 1977.*
45. Coccia PF, Kersey JH, Gajl-Peczalska KJ, *et al*: Prognostic significance of surface marker analysis in childhood non-Hodgkin's lymphoproliferative malignancies. *Am J Hematol 1:405–417, 1976.*
46. Jones SE, Fuks Z, Bull M, *et al*: Non-Hodgkin's lymphomas. IV. Clinicopathological correlation in 405 cases. *Cancer 31:806–823, 1973.*
47. Schein PS, Chabner BA, Canellos, GP, *et al*: Potential for prolonged disease-free survival following combination chemotherapy of non-Hodgkin's lymphoma. *Blood 43:181–189, 1974.*
48. Berard CW, Jaffe ES, Braylan RB, *et al*: Immunologic aspects and pathology of the malignant lymphomas. *Cancer 42:911–921, 1978.*
49. Lukes RJ, Collins RD: New observations on follicular lymphoma, in Akazaki K, Rappaport H, Berard CW, *et al* (eds): *Malignant Diseases of the Hematopoietic System. Gann Monograph on Cancer Research 15*. University Park Press, Baltimore, London, Tokyo, 1973, p. 209–215.
50. Garvin AJ, Simon RM, Jones R, *et al*: The National Cancer Institute experience with non-Hodgkin's lymphomas; a clinicopathologic review of 473 cases (abstract). *Lab Invest 40:255–256, 1979.*
51. Garvin AJ, Spicer SS, McKeever PE: The cytochemical demonstration of intracellular immunoglobulin; in neoplasms of lymphoreticular tissue. *Am J Pathol 82:457–478, 1976.*
52. Taylor CR: An immunohistological study of follicular lymphoma, reticulum cell sarcoma and Hodgkin's disease. *Eur J Cancer 12:61–75, 1976.*
53. Callihan TR, Braylan RB, Farnham R, *et al*: Correlation between immunohistochemistry and cell surface markers in diffuse large cell (''histiocytic'') lymphomas (abstract). *Lab Invest 40:244, 1979.*
54. Mann RB, Jaffe ES, Berard CW: Malignant lymphomas; a conceptual understanding of morphologic diversity. *Am J Pathol 94:105–192, 1979.*

CHAPTER THREE

Investigation of Non-Hodgkin's Lymphoma in Children by Surface Phenotyping Techniques

J. A. HABESHAW, PhD, MD

NON-HODGKIN'S LYMPHOMA (NHL) in children is a rare disease and appears in forms that are strikingly different from the adult counterpart. The most notable differences are the relative absence of nodular or follicular lymphomas in children, the high incidence of thymic tumors, the frequent association between lymphoma and acute leukemia, and the occurrence of malignant histiocytosis in contrast to its extreme rarity in adults. Because of the rarity of non-Hodgkin's lymphoma in children, few centers have enough data available to suggest new approaches to the histological and functional characterization of this disease.

In this chapter, 36 non-Hodgkin's lymphomas of childhood are examined by their surface phenotype and related to the Kiel histological classification.[1] The findings of other childhood series in the literature have also been reviewed. The results clearly show how childhood lymphoid malignancies differ from their adult counterparts, and suggest likely functional differences between the two groups.

THE RELEVANCE OF THE CELL PHENOTYPE TO THE INVESTIGATION OF LYMPHOMA

Establishing the phenotype of a malignant cell allows that cell to be allocated (1) to a discrete class on the basis of class-specific phenotypic features, and (2) to a subclass on the basis of other phenotypic features that are not class specific but may be linked to differentiation or maturation.[2] This results in a complete description of the malignancy, and enables other malignancies of similar phenotype to be related

Department of Medical Oncology, St. Bartholomew's Hospital, West Smithfield, London, EC1A 7BE, England

to it. Surface phenotyping is an essential component of any current study of non-Hodgkin's lymphomas.

Class-specific phenotypic features

The expression of a class-specific phenotypic feature defines the class of cell to which the cell expressing it belongs. Several examples are known and these will be described.

The ALL antigen is a cell-class-specific antigen expressed on lymphomyeloid cells at an early stage in their differentiation. The class defined by ALL-antigen expression may be the lymphomyeloid stem cell, since these cells occur only in bone marrow, and malignancies expressing ALL antigen are all acute leukemias/lymphomas of lymphoblastic type or occur during lymphoblastic crisis of chronic granulocytic leukemia.[3] Several subclasses of ALL-antigen-positive cells exist, including the precursor cell of the B-lymphoid line (pre-B cell).[4]

T lymphocytes exhibit two class-specific features: the expression of the human T-lymphocyte antigen (HTLA) system and the capacity to detect and proliferate in response to HLA antigen differences in mixed lymphocyte culture. Cells that express human T-lymphocyte antigen may nonetheless be immunologically incompetent, such as prothymocytes of the bone marrow, and cannot be said to be "differentiated" in terms of function. Human T-lymphocyte antigen expression defines the T-lymphocyte class irrespective of the degree of functional maturity of T cell.[5]

B lymphocytes express surface immunoglobulin, which is synthesized by the cell. Synthesis of immunoglobulin is a class-specific feature of B lymphocytes, and its expression on the cell surface coincides with the functional definition of B cell immunocompetence.[6] The hypervariable regions of the expressed immunoglobulin molecule provide the antigen receptor that mediates the B cell response to antigen.

Differentiation or maturation linked phenotypic features

The Ia-like antigen (gp 28/33) is a glycoprotein expressed on most ALL-positive stem cells, on B cells and suppressor T cells, and weakly on immature myeloid cells.[7] Since its expression is not restricted to one cell class, it is not a class-specific antigen. The expression of Ia antigen may be linked to differentiation or maturation, since on myeloid cells it becomes more weakly expressed as the cell matures and is not present on granulocytes. It is apparently expressed only on postthymic (?suppressor) T cell subsets, and not on cortical thymocytes or prethymic T cells. It is also expressed on most B cells,[8] but may be absent from plasma cells.

The enzyme terminal deoxynucleotidyl transferase (TdT)[9-11] is also a differentiation-linked rather than class-specific phenotypic marker. This enzyme polymerizes nucleotide phosphate bases onto single stranded DNA without a template. TdT enzyme activity is limited in tissue distribution to bone marrow and thymic cortex. In bone marrow, ALL-antigen-positive stem cells, as well as the pre-B cells, are TdT positive. Prethymic and thymic T cell subsets are TdT positive. All B cells positive for surface immunoglobulin (SIg), differentiated myeloid cells (granulocytes and mononuclear phagocytes), and postthymic (i.e., functionally immunocompetent) T cells are TdT negative. TdT activity can be said to identify all classes of functionally incompetent, and therefore undifferentiated, lymphomyeloid cells.[12]

The receptors for complement and the Fc portion of IgG (Fcγ, Fcμ, C3B/C4b, C3d) are expressed by cells of more than one class. The expression of these receptors is probably of functional significance, controlling T and B cell interaction, triggering, and maturation of immunologically competent T and B cells. An example is the restricted expression of Fcμ receptors to T cell subsets with helper function[13] and Fcγ receptors to suppressor T cells.[14,15] The Fcμ receptor is also present on (only) a restricted subset of immature B cells. In addition, C3d receptor expression, without the C3b receptor, characterizes the B cell population of the lymph node germinal follicle.[16]

On the basis of these phenotypic markers, it is possible to identify subclasses of undifferentiated and differentiated lymphoid cells, which can be related to the known subsets of lymphocytes. The subsets identified are shown in Tables 1, 2, and 3.

T cell subsets

In humans, T cells exhibiting TdT and HTLA positivity but lacking E receptors occur in some forms of ALL.[17] E-rosetting capacity is gained in the thymus. Human T-lymphocyte antigens form a group of seven antigenic specificities, two of which are glycoprotein, and a further one, which is expressed only on thymic lymphocytes.[18] Subsets of peripheral and thymic T cells have been found expres-

TABLE 1
Undifferentiated or Functionally Incompetent Lymphoid Cells

Cell type	Probable origin	Phenotype
Lymphomyeloid stem cell	Marrow	ALL+ Ia+ TdT+
Pre-B cell	Marrow Fetal liver	ALL+ Ia+ TdT±– Cytoplasmic μ chain+
Pre-T cell	Marrow	HTLA+ E rosette– TdT+
Cortical thymocyte	Thymic cortex	HTLA+ E rosette+ TdT+
Fetal thymocyte	Fetal thymus	HTLA+ E rosette+ TdT±– C3d+

TABLE 2
Differentiated T-Lymphocyte Subsets

Cell type	Probable origin	Phenotype
Medullary thymocyte	Thymic Medulla	HTLA+ E rosette+ Fcγ+ Fcμ+ TdT–
Peripheral T cell	Node Spleen	HTLA+ E rosette+ TdT–
T (helper)	Node Spleen Blood	HTLA+ E rosette+ Fcμ+ TdT–
T (suppressor)	Blood Node Spleen	HTLA+ E rosette+ Fcγ+ TdT– Ia+

TABLE 3
Differentiated B-Lymphocyte Subsets

Cell type	Probable origin	Phenotype
Immature B(1)	Marrow Blood Spleen	Ia+ weak SIgM+ TdT–
Immature B(2)	Marrow Blood Spleen	Ia+ weak SIgM+ Fcμ+ Fcγ+
Immature B(3)	Marrow Blood Spleen	Ia+ weak SIgM+ Fcμ+ Fcγ+ C3d+ (C3b+)
Primary response B cell	Marrow Spleen	Ia+ SIgM+ CyIgM+
Primary response B lymphoblast	Marrow Spleen	Ia+ SIgM+ CyIgM+ (Noncapping SIg)
Follicular B cell	Node Tonsil Peyer's patch	Ia+ SIgM+ C3d+
B Immunoblast	Node	Ia+ SIgM+G or SIgG+ (Noncapping SIg)
"Memory" B cell	Blood Spleen	Ia+ SIg+ Fcγ+ C3d+ (C3b+)
Proplasma cell	Node Peyer's patch	SIgM or M+G or G+ or A+ CyIgG/A+
Plasma cell	Node	SIg– CyIg+ (?Ia–)

sing Fcγ and Fcμ and C3 receptors alone or in combination.[19-21] Among these subsets, fetal thymocytes have been described with the phenotype E or E− C3d+ + TdT±.[12,22] The fact that Fcγ and Fcμ receptor expression by peripheral T cells can be modulated by exposure to γ- or μ-containing immune complexes[23] suggests that either helper or suppressor subsets could be derived from an Fcγ- and Fcμ-positive precursor.

B cell subsets

The B cell system in man is rather more difficult to analyze. While T cell development is independent of antigen stimulation, B cell development is controlled largely by the "antigen drive," which stimulates proliferation and selective elimination of B cell precursors. The resulting B cell population is determined by the antigenic "history" of the individual from which it is derived. As a result, B cell populations are more heterogenous than T cell populations, making the interpretation of the phenotypic features of B cells less precise than that of T cells.

B cells are derived from the pre-B precursor (ALL+ Ia+ TdT+ Cyμ chain+), which has been described in fetal liver and bone marrow in humans and in murine species.[2,4,24,25] The immature B cell expresses surface IgM rather weakly, and is easily "tolerized" or blockaded by the administration of a specific antigen or anti-μ chain antisera.[26] Studies in mice clearly show that the immature B cell acquires Fcγ receptor before C3 receptor.[27] In humans, immature B cell subsets are rarely a major part of the B cell population except in the neonatal period. In the adult, most B cells are derived from populations of memory, follicular, or pro-plasma cells already committed to an immune response. Immature B cells may form a component of tumors of young children or may be seen in chronic lymphocytic leukemia of adults, particularly when the disease is restricted to bone marrow and spleen. The pre-B cell is cytologically distinct from the other Cy Ig+ cell classes and is isomorphic with undifferentiated cells of ALL.

The selection of antigen-responsive B cells occurs in two stages, and only selected subsets form a significant part of the B cell population in the adult. The first stage is the primary immune response, where "virgin" B cells are converted to IgM-secreting cells. IgM antibody-antigen immune complex so formed may exert further selection pressure on clones of follicular B cell precursors as they develop in the germinal center. Complement and IgM antibody are known to influence germinal center formation.[28,29] Bone marrow precursors of germinal center B cells are of unknown phenotype. The experimental study of germinal center development in rabbits shows that bone marrow precursors migrate to, and proliferate in, the germinal center, and that the resulting memory cell population migrates to spleen or to the lymphocyte corona around already existing germinal centers.[30,31] Most germinal center B cells die during their rapid proliferative phase, but those which produce high affinity antigen receptors remain viable, and survive as memory cells or plasma cell precursors. The formation of germinal follicles, and the subsequent conversion of postfollicular B cells to antibody secreting cells requires T cell help.[32,33]

In tonsil, antigen-reactive cells proliferate under the stimulus of locally fixed antigen, to produce follicular B cells of SIg+ C3d+ phenotype. From these cells are derived precursors of the "memory" cell and plasma cell. The conversion of the postfollicular B cell to the antibody-forming plasma cell involves the suppression of SIg, Fc, and C3 receptor expression, probably loss of Ia antigen, immunoglobulin "switching" from M to G heavy chain, and the development of plasma-cell-specific antigens.[34-38] The plasma cell derived from the IgM-secretory phase of a primary immune response differs from the IgG-secreting plasma cell of a secondary response in that cytoplasmic IgM-positive cells usually retain some SIg expression, while IgG-secreting (or IgA-secreting) plasma cells are commonly SIg negative.

PREPARATION AND USE OF SURFACE MARKERS

Antisera currently available for detection of ALL, HTLA, Ia, and myeloid antigens have been adequately described in the literature.[2,3,7,8,18] These antisera are used as fluorescein-labelled $F(ab')_2$ fragments or in sandwich immunofluorescence tests. Their use is essential in defining the subclasses of non-Hodgkin's lymphoma in children, because many of the lesions do not express other markers such as SIg or E-rosetting. Heteroantisera all suffer from the disadvantage that the defined specificities are dependent on the range of antigens to which the immunized rabbit will respond. Most of these antigens will be species specific (i.e., antihuman) rather than anticell specific. In addition, the activity of the absorbed antiserum depends greatly upon the extent of absorption, and the phenotypic class of cells used for that absorption. These difficulties are likely to be overcome when monoclonal antibodies derived from hybridomas become more readily available.

Antisera against heavy chains (M,D,A,G, and E) and light chains (k and λ) are commercially available. They are specific, but specific antibody is often present in low titer. Further purification by immunoabsorbent columns or the use of defined batches of antiserum of high titer is necessary to avoid cross reactions when used on cell suspensions. Antisera can be used in the form of $F(ab')_2$ fragments to avoid nonspecific binding to Fc receptors, or the antisera must be prepared aggregate-free by centrifugation at 110,000 *g* for 1 h before use. Sandwich techniques are more sensitive than direct immunofluorescence for detecting surface immunoglobulin. They have the additional advantage of rapidly capping some lymphocytes, thus distinguishing them from noncapping B cells (usually lymphoblasts or immunoblasts).

For the detection of cytoplasmic μ chain in the pre-B cells, purified antihuman rabbit μ-chain antibody is used as a rhodamine conjugate. In this technique, cells are stained for SIg with fluorescein isothiocyanate conjugate (FITC), cytocentrifuged, and stained for intracellular μ chain with the rhodamine conjugate.

The techniques of E-rosetting are well known. Those using a preincubation of cells at 37°C, followed by pelleting and incubation for 1–2 h at 4°C or 20°C are more sensitive than the "active" rosette test. Fc receptors for IgG and IgM (Fcγ, Fcμ) are detected in a rosette test using ox red cells, which have two advantages over sheep red cells. The ox red cells (1) are less agglutinable, and so can be more heavily sensitized than sheep cells, and (2) form very few spontaneous rosettes with T or B cells.

The receptor for complement most commonly detected is the C3d receptor, using IgM-sensitized red cells incubated with mouse serum or human R3 reagent. Pure reagents for detection of C3b/C4b are difficult to prepare since they require purified complement components for their manufacture. The expression of E, Fcγ, Fcμ, and C3d receptors by tumor cells are important features of the various subclasses defined by class-specific antisera, TdT activity, SIg, CyIg, and Ia antigen expression. The proper study of a lymphoid cell population requires that all of these features should be examined in every case. The method of choice for the study of lymphomas is to mark the cells present in a viable cell suspension. Counting the percentages of cells expressing each marker provides a profile of the tumor. The cells may also be identified in frozen section using class-specific antisera. The cytology of rosette-forming cells can be determined from good cytocentrifuge preparations. The expression of surface immunoglobulin must be determined after stripping cell-bound immunoglobulin and immune complexes from the cell surface. This is achieved (1) by trypsinization followed by culture to allow resynthesis of immunoglobulin, or (2) by washing in acetate buffer at pH 5.5, which effectively displaces bound complexes from the lymphocyte surface without affecting membrane immunoglobulin.

The study of normal tissues from children shows that lymphoid populations exhibit quite marked phenotypic variability, particularly in the peripheral lymph nodes. In Tables 4 and 5, values are given for some "normal" nodes, reactive nodes, and thymus glands. In Tables 4–10, results for each immunological marker are expressed as percent of positive cells.

HISTOLOGICAL AND PHENOTYPIC CORRELATES IN CHILDHOOD NON-HODGKIN'S LYMPHOMA

The histological appearances of non-Hodgkin's lymphomas in children are quite different from those of adults. The classification used in this presentation is Lennert's (1978) modification of the Kiel classification.[39] In the material he presents, Lennert finds that non-Hodgkin's lymphomas in children can usually be classified as (1) lymphoblastic, in which he defines three subgroups: lymphoblastic lymphoma of null cells, lymphoblastic lymphoma of T cell type, and lymphoblastic lymphoma of B cells (divided into Burkitt's (EBNA+) and non-Burkitt's (EBNA−) tumors); (2) immunoblastic tumors; (3) centroblastic tumors; and (4) malignant histiocytosis. In the unmodified Rappaport scheme[40] most of the lymphoblastic tumors would be classified as diffuse poorly differentiated lymphocytic lymphomas. In more recent classifications, many of these would now be

TABLE 4
Normal and Reactive Lymph Node Profiles in Children

Site	Age	E	Fcγ	Fcμ	C3d	SIg	Phagocytes	Condition
Neck	10	59	25	2	28	30	4	Reactive
Splenic hilum	12	62	38	6	34	27	1	Spherocytosis
Neck	12	70	8	2	24	25	3	Follicular hyperplasia
Mesenteric	11	21	20	14	26	36	2	"Normal"
Neck	4 mo.	67	59	13	46	22	4	Reactive
Inguinal	16	55	18	NA	40	32	7	Sinus hyperplasia
Mesenteric	10	38	13	NA	52	35	27	"Normal"
Mesenteric	10	50	45	22	41	22	3	"Normal"
Neck	8	18	7	4	2	50	7	Toxoplasmosis
Inguinal	12	56	29	NA	49	32	12	Reactive

TABLE 5
Immunological Reactivity of Thymus in Normal Full Term Infants and in Fetuses

Thymus of normal full term infants
Percentage of cells expressing E, Fcγ, Fcμ, C3d, and SIg

E	Fcγ	Fcμ	C3d	SIg
71	2	0	0	0
79	7	10	2	1
72	22	17	10	0
74	20	24	2	2
92	60	34	8	4

Fetal thymus
Percentage of cells expressing E, Fcγ, C3d, and SIg

Estimated gestational age	E	Fcγ	C3d	SIg
15-16 weeks	27	3	60	$<$1%
21-23 weeks	29	12	68	$\leqslant$1%

redefined as undifferentiated lymphocytic lymphomas. Centroblastic and immunoblastic tumors would probably be classified as diffuse histiocytic using the unmodified Rappaport scheme, and this group would also include malignant histiocytosis.

One of the peculiarities of non-Hodgkin's lymphomas in children is the frequent association between peripheral lymphadenopathy, thymic enlargement, and a leukemic blood picture. Many arguments about the distinction between ALL and lymphoblastic lymphoma can now be resolved on the basis of the phenotypic features. In most instances the phenotype of cells from lymphoblastic lymphoma, especially of T cell and null cell types, does not differ from the phenotype of the corresponding acute leukemia. Clinical distinctions between ALL and lymphoblastic lymphoma cannot in most cases be sustained on phenotypic grounds. Thymic lymphoblastic lymphomas appear to involve thymus and lymph nodes, with later involvement of the blood and bone marrow. In addition, the phenotypes of the neoplasm indicate an origin from functionally immature T lymphocytes, equivalent to those found in T cell ALL, which shows marrow involvement at the time of initial presentation. The prethymic T cell profile (E− HTLA+ TDT+) presents more frequently as acute leukemia than lymphoblastic lymphoma, although mediastinal and lymph node involvement can occur with this phenotype. Moreover, both B and T cell lymphoblastic lymphomas characteristically spread to the meninges, to the testes, and to the CSF, behavior that also characterizes T cell ALL.

In the B-lymphoblastic group the lymphoma rarely presents as a primary lymph node disease. Here the leukemic phase may be preceded by abdominal lymph node involvement, primary tumor of the bowel or extranodal massive deposits. The B-lymphoblastic tumors can also appear as SIg+ B cell ALL (rare) or as pre-B cell ALL (more common).

Lymphoblastic tumors: null cell lymphoblastic lymphomas

Lymphoblastic lymphomas of non-B, non-T type are formed from cells showing light to moderate cytoplasmic basophilia, granular PAS positivity, and negative acid phosphatase reactions. Phenotypically these cells express ALL and Ia antigen, are TdT positive, but do not react with HTLA antisera, are E-rosette and SIg negative, and do not express Fcγ, Fcμ, or C3d receptors. In most instances the cells lack evidence of cytoplasmic μ chain, but occasional cases, possibly 15–20% of ALL+ malignancies, are of pre-B cell type (Cy μ chain positive).[41] Lennert distinguishes in this group two forms of tumor. In the first form, the presentation is that of acute lymphoblastic leukemia, in which invasion and destruction of lymph nodes and extranodal tissues is minimal. In the second form, the presentation is more in keeping with lymphoma, with extensive lymph node involvement, local infiltration and tissue destruction, and late marrow involvement. The second type is subclassified as "lymphoblastic sarcoma," and the first type is classified as lymphoblastic malignancy of undifferentiated type.

T-lymphoblastic lymphomas

Lymphoblastic lymphomas of T cell type usually affect an older age group (11–16 years) than lymphoblastic lymphoma of undifferentiated type (2–10 years) and are more common in boys. The tumor is composed of moderately basophilic lymphoblasts, showing focal acid phosphatase positivity. The cells are frequently of smaller size than in B or null cell lymphoblastic lymphoma, and many show convoluted nuclei (best seen in good cytocentrifuge preparations). Mediastinal mass occurs commonly with supraclavicular lymph node enlargement and pleural effusion. Phenotypically the cells are HTLA+, E rosette+, and many express C3d receptors. Most, but not all, cases are TdT positive. These tumors frequently become leukemic, although gross marrow involvement is not always present at diagnosis, and meningeal involvement may also occur. As mentioned, in most instances the distinction between this subgroup of lymphoma and T cell ALL is blurred. Pre-T cell lymphoblastic leukemias and lymphomas are more commonly classified cytologically as ALL or as undifferentiated (phenotype E− HTLA+ TdT+), since they lack the convoluted nucleus of the thymic lymphocyte (phenotype E+ HTLA+ TdT+), although they usually show weak acid phosphatase positivity.

B-lymphoblastic lymphomas

Lymphoblastic lymphomas of B cell type are composed of cells with strongly basophilic cytoplasm, exhibiting PAS positivity. The peak age of presentation is between three and seven years. Three cytological types are described: (1) Burkitt's tumors, which are Epstein-Barr nuclear antigen positive (EBNA+), are composed of small cells resembling centroblasts, with deeply basophilic cytoplasm, often with cytoplasmic vacuolation, and showing the "starry sky" appearance due to irregularly distributed macrophages in lymph node sections. They lack acid phosphatase activity, and are α-napthyl esterase negative and strongly pyroninophilic. The cells are more cohesive than either the centroblast or the undifferentiated lymphoblast. Lennert favors an origin from germinal center cells, probably centroblasts, rather than from undifferentiated lymphoblasts, although sections of undifferentiated lymphomas may also show the "starry sky" appearance.[39] (2) B cell lymphoblastic lymphomas of non-Burkitt type (EBNA−) occur in children and adults. These tumors are similar in histological appearance to the Burkitt tumor. The cytological features are equivalent to those of known cases of EBNA+ tumors. (3) B cell ALL is very uncommon, but lymph node involvement can occur, and mediastinal and pleural involvement is not unknown in this disease.

Immunoblastic tumors

Immunoblastic malignancies occur with greater frequency in adults than in children, the median age of presentation being 63 years. Both B cell- and T cell-derived immunoblastic malignancies can occur, but the majority are of B cell type. The cells are large and basophilic, and the nucleoli are large and well defined. Moderate amounts of cytoplasm are present. Giant cells may occur, and some tumors are markedly pleomorphic. The categorization of a tumor as B immunoblastic depends upon the demonstration of elevated immunoglobulin levels in the affected node, and malignant plasmablasts (SIg− CyIg+) form a variable component of the lesion.

In previous histological classifications, immunoblastic lymphoma was classified as diffuse histiocytic lymphoma or as reticulosarcoma. This group also contains tumors composed of cells that are morphologically immunoblasts, but which do not show surface immunoglobulin or HTLA positivity. These cells are not phenotypically equivalent to the ALL+ lymphoblast since they are ALL−, and the term "receptor silent" has been used to describe them. They resemble plasmablastic lymphoma in their surface phenotype, but lack cytoplasmic immunoglobulin. The phenotype of immunoblastic B cell tumors shows that SIg expression is strong, but remains distributed as stippled patches on the cell surface when stained with FITC labelled anti-Ig antisera. Capping of surface immunoglobulin antiimmunoglobulin complex is not seen, even after prolonged incubation at 37°C.

Centroblastic tumors

Centroblastic lymphomas are rare in children. They commonly resemble the lymphoblastic lymphoma of Burkitt's type and can show the characteristic starry sky appearance. In our own series of adult lymphomas,[42] centroblastic tumors were commonly composed of T lymphocytes with an associated B-lymphoid component expressing monoclonal immunoglobulin. No examples of this tumor class have so far been seen in this study in children, and the phenotype of childhood centroblastic tumor is unknown.

PHENOTYPIC VARIANTS IN THE PRESENT SERIES

Lymphoblastic lymphomas of null cell (undefined) type

Lymph node tumors were classified as lymphoblastic lymphomas of null cell type if they showed (1) lymphoblastic histology/cytology, (2) ALL-antigen expression, (3) TdT positivity, and (4) nonexpression of Fcγ, Fcμ, C3d, SIg, or CyIg markers. Seven tumors of this class were seen, six in boys and one in a girl. The median age of presentation was 5 years (range 3–16 years). Similar tumors have been seen in patients up to 20 years of age. The profiles of the affected lymph nodes are shown in Table 6. Medians of less than 10% were seen for each marker. Functional phagocytes formed less than 1% in each case. In all tested cases, the cells were ALL+ and Ia+. HTLA-positive cells were confined to the E-rosetting population. All patients had bone marrow involvement, elevated leukocyte counts, with ALL+ Ia+ blast cells in the circulation. In no case was cytoplasmic μ chain detected. These tumors are regarded as variants of ALL.

TABLE 6
Lymph Node Profiles in Malignant Lymphoma,
Lymphoblastic Null Cell Type (ALL+ Ia+ TdT+)

	Age	Sex	E	Fcμ	Fcγ	C3d	Phagocytes	SIg
	3	F	3	3	1	5	<1	6
	16	M	4	3	0	0	<1	10
	6	M	5	1	12	17	0	21
	4	M	8	0	3	3	0	1[a]
	4	M	20	0	1	17	0	11
	11	M	2	1	1	8	0	0
	6	M	2	4	7	2	0	0
Medians	6		4	1	1	5	0	6

[a]ALL, TdT not tested.

Lymphoblastic lymphomas of T cell type

Tumors of T cells were studied in 10 patients under the age of 16 years (Table 7). All showed the characteristic morphology/cytology of T cell-lymphoblastic lymphomas, including convoluted nucleus and acid phosphatase positivity. Seven patients were leukemic at diagnosis, two of the remaining three developed leukemia during the course of the disease. The criteria for inclusion in this category were (1) lymphoblastic histology/cytology with acid phosphatase positivity, and (2) predominance of E-rosette-positive and HTLA-positive cells. The ages ranged from 4 to 15 years with a median of 11 years. Three patients were girls and seven were boys. Phenotyping distinguished the following groups: E− HTLA+ TdT+ (1 case), E+ HTLA+ TdT+ (6 cases), E+ C3d+ TdT− (2 cases), and E− HTLA+ C3d+ TdT+ (1 case).

The case showing the E− HTLA+ TdT+ profile occurred in a male child four years of age. Only 21% of cells were E+, but 75% were HTLA+. ALL and Ia antigens were not present. TdT levels were elevated at 27 units/10^8 cells (normal <5 units). SIg+ B cells comprised 29% of the tumor population, and these expressed no C3d or Fc receptors. The SIg expression was polyclonal. The cases of E+ HTLA+ TdT+ phenotype occurred in children aged 9 to 15 years. E rosettes were formed on 62–91% of the cells present, and these cells were also HTLA positive. From 0 to 11% of cells were SIg positive. Fcμ (1–10%), Fcγ (1–3%), and C3d (1–3%) receptor expression was negative in all cases. TdT varied between 17 and 95.5 units/10^8 cells.

Three cases showed the presence of C3d receptor as well as E receptor or HTLA positivity on the tumor cells. In the first case, a boy of four years, the node biopsy

TABLE 7
Malignant Lymphoma Lymphoblastic T Cell Type (HTLA Positive)

	Age	Sex	E	Fcγ	Fcμ	C3d	Phagocytes	SIg	TdT
	12	M	91	5	1	1	<1	0	+
	15	M	87	0	0	0	<1	2	+
	11	M	46	1	10	2	0	0	+
	14	F	36	1	1	1	0	0	+
	7	M	62	1	1	3	1	6	+
	9	F	73	3	2	3	0	11	+
	4	M	21	3	1	1	0	29	+
	7	M	39	14	1	39	0	13	+
	11	F	70	40	0	58	10	12	ND
(a)	4	M	71	16	24	26	2	15	−
(b)	5	M	73	2	3	64	1	12	−
Medians	9		70	3	1	3	<1	11	

showed 70% of E+ HTLA+ cells with Fcγ 16%, Fcμ 24%, C3d 26%, and SIg+ cells 15%. The presentation was of mediastinal and supraclavicular lymph node enlargement, with a pleural effusion. The cells in a recurrence of the pleural effusion removed 275 days after the initial biopsy showed 73% E-rosette-positive T cells, with Fcγ 2%, Fcμ 3%, and C3d receptor 64% positive. Both node and effusion were TdT negative (<5 units/10^8 cells). Cytocentrifuge preparations clearly demonstrated C3d rosetting by T cells with typical convoluted nuclei. A supraclavicular node biopsy in an 11-year-old girl was of similar type, with 70% of cells E+, 40% Fcγ+, 0% Fcμ+, and 58% C3d+. TdT levels in this patient's node were not determined. The cytology was that of T cell-lymphoblastic lymphoma, with acid phosphatase positivity. In the final case, a boy seven years of age, the lymph node profile showed only 39% of cells E rosette positive, although 69% were HTLA+. Fcγ 14%, Fcμ 1%, C3d 39%, and SIg+ 13% constituted the remaining profile. In this case TdT levels were elevated (19.5 units/10^8 cells).

In this limited series, the heterogeneity of T cell-lymphoblastic malignancy is well illustrated, including one case of possible pre-T cell malignancy (E− HTLA+ TdT+) and five cases of E+ HTLA+ TdT+ tumor. Two of these tumors terminated fatally with CNS involvement, and both exhibited HTLA+ E+ TdT+ phenotypes. The patient with E+ C3d+ TdT− phenotype died with widespread disease 14 months from diagnosis.

Lymphoblastic lymphoma of B cell type

Eleven patients had lymphoblastic lymphomas of B cell type. Two of these patients had a tumor of the scalp. The median age was 6 years (range 6 months to 14 years). Seven were boys. In two patients cytoplasmic IgM immunoglobulin was present, in addition to surface IgM. Three patients showed a predominance of noncapping cells, including one with cytoplasmic IgM. Six of the B-lymphoblastic lymphomas expressed Fcγ, Fcμ, or C3d receptors on the B cells. The phenotypes were as follows: SIg+ CyIg+ (2 cases), SIg+ (3 cases), SIg+ Fcγ+ (2 cases), SIg+ C3d+ (4 cases) (Table 8).

In 4 of the 11 patients, abdominal masses were the primary site of the disease. Four patients expressed C3d receptors on more than 25% of tumor cells. One patient expressed Fcγ receptor on 43% of cells, and showed 16% of C3d receptors. In two patients, both G and M immunoglobulin heavy chains were present on the cell surface. Leukemic involvement of the marrow was present at diagnosis in five patients. Two of the 11 patients with B-lymphoblastic lymphoma have died within one year of diagnosis.

Immunoblastic lymphomas (ML IB)

Immunoblastic lymphomas were uncommon in this series, being diagnosed in only four patients. The profile of these tumors is shown in Table 9. Two of these tumors failed to show either T cell or B cell surface markers, did not react with anti-ALL

TABLE 8
Lymphoblastic Lymphoma of B Lymphocytes (All SIg Positive and TdT Negative)

Involved sites	Sex	Age	E	Fcγ	Fcμ	C3d	SIg	CyIg	Ig class	Comment
Marrow + node	M	3	6	8	18	13	80	++	Mk	Leukemic
Marrow + scalp	M	11	4	0	4	2	82	++	Mk	Leukemic
Marrow + scalp	F	6 mo.	0	1	0	0	78	–	Mk	Leukemic
Marrow + node	F	4	6	29	25	1	58	–	–[a]	Leukemic
Marrow + node	M	6	5	12	1	17	43	–	Mk	Leukemic
Abdominal mass	M	14	35	1	1	32	40	–	Mk	
Illiocecal mass	F	16	15	4	0	36	82	–	GMk	
Abdominal mass	M	8	29	8	0	45	58	–	Mk	
Abdominal mass	F	6	20	1	1	30	52	–	GMk	
Node	M	14	6	2	1	1	54	–	Mk	
Node	M	11	0	43	3	16	60	–	Mk	
Medians		8	6	4	1	16	58			

[a]Insufficient cells available for determination of Ig class.

TABLE 9
Surface Markers in Immunoblastic Lymphoma

Tissue	Age	Sex	Fcγ	Fcμ	C3D	SIg	CyIg	Ig Class
Node	4	M	1	1	17	10	Neg	Polyclonal
Rectal biopsy	4	M	1	2	15	0	Neg	
Postnasal space	8	F	15			59	ND	Mk
Tonsil	14	M	2	1	1	51	ND	Mk

antisera, and belong to the category defined as "receptor silent." The two B cell tumors exhibited noncapping surface immunoglobulin of the Mk class.

Malignant histiocytosis

Malignant histiocytosis involving lymph nodes is a rare condition in adults, even when associated with monocytic leukemia (Naegeli type). The Schilling type arises primarily in lymph nodes and is not associated with early bone marrow and blood involvement; it has been seen only once in over 150 adult biopsies. Subgroups of malignant disease of the mononuclear phagocyte system can now be defined by cytochemistry and surface phenotyping. More important, the use of surface marking shows that many so-called histiocytic tumors are of B cell derivation and that, of the remainder, relatively few show the florid phenotypic and functional characteristics of histiocytes (macrophages) such as Fcγ, C3d receptors and phagocytosis. Cytochemistry shows mononuclear phagocytes to contain large amounts of acid phosphatase, nonspecific ASD acetate esterase, ASD chloracetate esterase and lysozyme. However, it is becoming apparent that not all tumors termed histiocytic have this histochemical profile or the phenotypic or functional features of mononuclear phagocytes. Histological evidence of phagocytosis is said to be a diagnostic feature of malignant histiocytosis, but it can occur in some subclasses of B cell lymphomas.

In this childhood series, four cases were classified as malignant histiocytosis on cytochemistry and cytology. Histology showed tumor cells of large size with oval nuclei and evidence of phagocytic potential. Three of the cases reported here would be classified as malignant histiocytosis on these criteria. In the fourth case, cells were obtained from the marrow of a child aged four months. In three of the four cases marrow was involved at diagnosis. The phenotype of these four tumors is shown in Table 10. They showed elevated levels of functional phagocytes, with substantial numbers of Fc and C3d receptors and of SIg-positive cells, though in only two was SIg expression judged to be monoclonal, and in all specimens, a minority of cells expressed these surface markers.

TABLE 10
Receptor Profile in Malignant Histiocytosis

Age	Sex	E	Fcγ	C3d	Phago-cytes	SIg	Ig class	Tissues involved
11	F	16	48	15	24	24	Polyclonal	Skin/node
9	M	13	27	13	16	14	IgDλ	Bone marrow, pleura, node
6 mo.	F	4	14	23	23	27	K	Node/marrow
4 mo.	F	5	32	21	22	15	Polyclonal	Marrow

In the two patients with possible monoclonal B cell populations, one showed the presence of IgDλ on the surface and in the cytoplasm of a substantial number of tumor cells. Serum IgD levels were not elevated. In the other patient, the SIg+ B cell population was distinct cytologically from the neoplastic "histiocytic" component of the lesion.

COMPARISON OF PHENOTYPIC CHARACTERISTICS OF NON-HODGKIN'S LYMPHOMA IN CHILDREN AND ADULTS

In a series of 115 adult lymphomas (aged more than 16 years) studied by the same methods, only eight examples of lymphoblastic lymphoma were seen. Three were of T cell type, two were ALL antigen positive, and three were of B cell type. Four of the five patients with T cell or ALL+ lymphoblastic lymphoma were under 32 years of age. Patients with B cell-lymphoblastic lymphoma were aged 55, 65, and 75 years, respectively. Thus lymphoblastic lymphoma is predominantly a disease of the child and young adult. In 115 lymph node biopsies in adults, the most common histological class was centroblastic and centrocytic tumor of both follicular and diffuse type (56 cases). Centrocytic tumors of both small and large cell type accounted for 12 cases, lymphocytic lymphoma for 10 cases, lymphoplasmacytoid (immunocytic) lymphoma for 9 cases, and centroblastic lymphoma accounted for 4 cases. Immunoblastic lymphoma was diagnosed on 16 occasions, and of these 2 were of receptor silent profile, two were of T cell, and 12 were of B cell phenotype. Only one case of malignant histiocytosis was diagnosed.

The histological categories in common between the adult and childhood series (lymphoblastic lymphoma, immunoblastic lymphoma, and malignant histiocytosis) formed only 24% of adult lymphomas. Categories not seen in children (centroblastic and centrocytic, lymphocytic and lymphoplasmacytoid tumor) formed almost 70% of adult lymphomas. A few tumors known to occur in both children and adults (e.g., centroblastic malignancies) were not found in the 36 cases of childhood non-Hodgkin's lymphoma examined. It is also known that nodular tumors (nodular poorly differentiated lymphoma, NPDL, of Rappaport) occasionally occur in children, but none were seen in this series.

On the basis of histological examination, we conclude: (1) lymphoblastic tumors of ALL+ cells or of T cells are from 7 to 10 times more frequent in children than in adults, (2) immunoblastic tumors of B cell or receptor-silent type occur with approximately equal frequency in the two groups, and (3) tumors classified as malignant histiocytosis may be 10 times more frequent in children. Obviously with the small numbers of cases examined, these data may be accurate. However, the trend is quite clear and emphasizes once again the reasons for the marked clinical and therapeutic differences between these groups.

On assessment of surface phenotype, 28% of childhood lymphomas were T cell derived, compared with only 5% of adult lymphomas (including immunoblastic lymphomas of T cells seen only in adults). The great majority of adult lymphomas were of B cell type (94 out of 115), and the most common phenotype was SIg+ C3d+ (35 cases), with SIg+ (25 cases) only slightly less common. Noncapping SIg+(19 cases), SIg+ Fcγ+ C3d+ (10 cases), and SIg+ CyIg+ (four cases) phenotypes formed the remaining variants of adult non-Hodgkin's lymphomas. The phenotypes SIg+ Fcγ+ Fcμ+ and SIg+ Fcγ+ Fcμ+ C3d+ were found only in cases of chronic lymphocytic leukemia. In childhood non-Hodgkin's lymphomas, B cell tumors were found in 11 cases (39%). As in adult lymphoma, the most common phenotype was of SIg+ C3d+ cells (four cases) with SIg+ (three cases), noncapping SIg+ (two cases), SIg+ CyIg+ (two cases, including one with noncapping cells), and two patients showing Fcγ+ SIg+ cells as the major phenotypic class in the tumor. The B cell subsets in non-Hodgkin's lymphoma in children do seem to differ in some respects from adult NHL. The frequency of SIg+ CyIg+ B cells is somewhat higher in children (approximately 20% in children and only 3% in adults). Few adult tumors with SIg+ Fcγ+ phenotype have been seen, although in chronic lymphocytic leukemia the phenotype SIg+ Fcγ+ Fcμ+ does occur. Noncapping SIg+ tumors and SIg+ C3d+ tumors occur in about equal frequency in adult and childhood non-Hodgkin's lymphomas.

ALL-antigen-positive tumors are much more common in children than in adults, where only three cases of ALL+ lymphoblastic lymphoma were seen. The receptor-silent tumors of both adults and children probably occur with similar frequency. In adults, these tumors are often abdominal or extranodal in origin, arising in gut-associated lymphoid tissue.

The phenotypic variants of T cell tumor in children are not unique. Pre-T cell ALL has been described in adults and E+ HTLA+ TdT+ lymphoma can occur.

CONCLUSIONS AND DISCUSSION OF THE NATURE OF NON-HODGKIN'S LYMPHOMA IN CHILDREN

The current literature on surface phenotyping in non-Hodgkin's lymphoma in children stresses the relationship between acute lymphoblastic leukemia and lymphoma in this age group. In a study of 49 cases of NHL in children,[43] the majority (36 out of 49) had ALL of undefined cell type (i.e., non-B, non-T). None of these patients had either mediastinal mass or abdominal node enlargement. Interestingly, in this group some cases with PAS-positive ALL cells showed enhanced C3 rosetting (sheep E, C3d). This subgroup may resemble the "fetal" thymic T cell cases described in this chapter, which were E− TdT±− C3d receptor positive, or these cases may be examples of prethymic T cell ALL. Seven out of 49 cases were of convoluted nucleated cells, of which 6 showed mediastinal involvement and 5 had a leukemic blood picture. Two of these cases showed the phenotype E+ C3+, one was E− C3d+, and five cases showed low levels of E rosetting (E−). Five cases showed acid phosphatase positivity. In 6 out of 49 cases classified as "small noncleaved follicular center cell" lymphoma/leukemia [which in the Kiel classification would correspond to ML LB (B)], all presented with abdominal symptoms. Four out of the six were leukemic and all were SIg positive, expressing both G and M heavy chain on the tumor cells with polyclonal light chain expression.

In a similar group of nine lymphoblastic malignancies of both children and adults examined,[44] no case expressed surface immunoglobulin, eight out of nine cases had a mediastinal mass, and five cases were TdT positive. Five cases also expressed E receptors on at least 20% of the cells. These authors conclude that lymphoblastic lymphomas are usually of T cell derivation. In 73 cases of non-Hodgkin's lymphoma studied by Coccia *et al.*,[45] seven patients had B cell lymphoblastic tumors (two of which showed E+ C3d+ phenotype), 13 had T cell tumors, and 53 patients had non-B non-T ALL-like malignancies, with a leukemic blood picture and relatively few "massive," i.e., tumorous lesions. The prognosis for T and B cell malignancies was notably worse than that of non-B non-T cell malignancy. In a report[46] of bone marrow involvement in Burkitt's lymphoma (lymphoblastic lymphoma of B cell type), 11 out of 13 patients described were less than 16 years old. Three out of four patients examined for surface phenotype had $\mu\lambda$ monoclonal SIg, and one patient had μk SIg.

In studies of terminal deoxynucleotidyl transferase (TdT) expression in lymphoid malignancy,[47] six cases of T cell lymphoblastic lymphoma were described as positive. One was E− C3+ TdT+, three were E+ TdT+, and two were E+ C3d+ TdT+. All of these patients were over 16 years of age. In a similar study of TdT activity in leukemia and lymphoma,[48] nine patients with lymphoblastic leukemia showed TdT positivity by immunofluorescence and by biochemical assay. Of these, four showed low levels of E rosette positive cells (E− phenotype). Two cases showed a combined expression of E rosettes and C3d receptors (phenotype E+ C3d+) and three cases E− C3d+ phenotype.

In a recently published review of 100 cases of non-Hodgkin's lymphoma in children (less than 16 years old),[49] four distinct groups were identified. A major group of "null" or undifferentiated neoplasms, appearing as ALL, formed 56% of lymphomas, with a peak age of presentation at six years. These correspond to the tumors of ALL+ Ia+ phenotype reported in this chapter. A second group of myeloid malignancies, again with leukemic presentation and characteristic features of acute myeloid leukemia, were found. Similar cases seen at this Unit have been excluded from the series reported here. T cell-lymphoblastic lymphoma/leukemia formed 14% of the cases. These showed lymphoblastic cytology, with frequent mediastinal involvement and extranodal spread, and had a poor prognosis. B cell-lymphoblastic lymphoma/leukemia showed Burkitt-like features and abdominal masses. In most cases the cells expressed SIg of monoclonal type with μ heavy chain the predominant heavy chain class. In a study of 23 children,[50] 22 of whom had acute lymphoblastic leukemia and one of whom had lymphoblastic lymphoma, three phenotypes were described: (1) null cell (E− C3−), (2) E+ C3+, and (3) E+ C3−. The phenotype E+ C3d+ has been called by these authors the "D" or doubly marked cell, and corresponds to the "fetal thymocyte" population described in this chapter. In another report, the conjunction of E and C3 receptors on the cells in a thymoma[51] were regarded as evidence of a "malignant" phenotype.

In two reviews of childhood lymphoma,[34,52] the major differences between adult and childhood non-Hodgkin's lymphomas are defined. Coccia[34] shows that the clinical behavior of lymphoid neoplasms in children is determined by the phenotypic characteristics of the blast cell, rather than the mode of presentation or the extent of marrow and blood involvement. He presents a strong case for regarding "null cell" and T cell lymphoma/leukemia as diseases in which a leukemic or nonleukemic presentation is irrelevant. In B cell lymphomas, Dehner[52] shows that Burkitt-like lymphoblastic tumors are more rarely leukemic than null cell or T cell tumors, but that they belong to a different class of B cell tumor than the common adult non-Hodgkin's lymphoma. Malignant histiocytosis is described as a lethal lymph node tumor in children that differs from lymphoblastic neoplasms of T, B, or null cell type. As shown in this chapter, malignant histiocytosis cells mark as "null" cells, although functional phagocytes also form part of the tumor. In histiocytic medullary reticulosis,[53] the tumor cells are described as functionally phagocytic and express C3 receptors, supporting the view that histiocytic tumors derived from the mononuclear phagocyte system do occur.

On the basis of published work, and the cases described in this chapter, it is possible to suggest a combined phenotypic and histological classification of childhood lymphoma/leukemia that indicates the likely histogenesis of each neoplasm. Tumors are classified on the basis of their phenotype primarily, since cells of the same phenotype must have a common origin irrespective of their histological appearance. The expression of subsidiary surface markers (Fcμ, Fcγ, C3d) may be important in determining the degree of functional differentiation of the tumor cell. This classification is given in Tables 11, 12, and 13, with only the groups affecting children shown.

In conclusion, the differences between adult and childhood lymphomas, when compared using phenotypic markers as the main criteria, show that the major adult classes are not represented in children. Most of the adult tumors are derived from functionally mature B cells of follicular or postfollicular origin. In contrast most

TABLE 11
Phenotypic Variants of Malignant Lymphoma Lymphoblastic Types (ML LB)

Phenotype	Probable cell or origin
Malignant lymphoma lymphoblastic undifferentiated (ALL)	
ALL+ Ia+ TdT+	Lymphomyeloid stem cell
ALL+ Ia+ TdT+ Cyμ chain+	Pre-B Cell
E– HTLA+ TdT+	Pre-T Cell
SIg+ (noncapping) (rare)	? Immature B Cell
Malignant lymphoma lymphoblastic (T) type	
E+ HTLA+ TdT+	Cortical thymocyte
E– HTLA+ TdT+ C3d+	Fetal thymocyte
E+ C3d+ TdT±	Fetal thymocyte
Malignant lymphoma lymphoblastic (B) type	
SIg+ CyIgM+	Primary response B lymphoblast
SIg+	Immature B cell
SIg+ Fcγ+ Fcμ±	Immature B cell
SIg+ C3d+	Follicular center Cell (centroblast or large centrocyte)

TABLE 12
Phenotypic Variants of Malignant Lymphoma Immunoblastic (ML IB) Type

Phenotype	Cell of origin
Noncapping SIg+	Immunoblast (primary or secondary immune response)
E+ HTLA+	T immunoblast
SIg– CyIg+	Plasmablast (secondary immune response)
SIg– E– HTLA– ALL– TdT–	Receptor silent cell (unknown origin)

TABLE 13
Phenotypic Variants of Malignant Histiocytosis

Phenotype	Probable origin
E– SIg– Fcγ+ C3d+	Monocyte (histiocyte)
E– SIg– Fcγ– C3d–	Unknown (receptor silent)
SIg+/E– SIg– Fc+ C3d+	Mixed B cell and histiocytic malignancy

tumors in children are of undifferentiated cells of stem cell or T cell class. The childhood T cell tumors show examples of prethymic and fetal thymic derivation, and mature T cell subset tumors of adults (T zone lymphomas) are not represented. B cell tumors of children show examples of primary immune response-derived B blasts, and B lymphoblastoid cells of follicular phenotype. Classical secondary immune response-derived immunoblastic or plasmablastic tumors are rare. Malignant tumors of phagocytes and receptor-silent cells are more common in children than in adults. The suggested phenotyping methods may serve in the future as a basis for clearly establishing the origins and biological behavior of childhood non-Hodgkin's lymphomas.

SUMMARY

The examination of lymphoma cells by surface marking techniques is a valuable aid to establishing the class of cell composing the tumor and serves as a guide to the degree of differentiation or maturation of that cell class. The resulting phenotype, when correlated with histological and cytological features, assists in establishing subdivisions of tumors that differ phenotypically while being isomorphous in histological or cytological appearance.

In a series of 36 cases of childhood non-Hodgkin's lymphoma, the phenotype of the neoplastic cells indicated heterogeneity in all the histologically defined categories. Lymphoblastic lymphoma of undifferentiated type probably consists of four phenotypically defined subclasses (stem cell, pre-T cell, pre-B cell, and immature B cell). Lymphoblastic lymphoma of T cell type has at least three phenotypic variants (thymic cortical T cells and fetal T cells). B lymphoblastic lymphomas have at least four main phenotypic variants (primary immune response lymphoblast, immature B cells of two types, and lymphoblasts of germinal follicle derivation).

In the category of immunoblastic malignancy, immunoblastic tumors of B cell and receptor-silent cell type were identified. Malignant histocytosis showed three phenotypic variants. On the basis of this limited study, a scheme indicating the phenotypic subtypes of childhood non-Hodgkin's lymphoma, their relationship to histology, and their probable cellular origins is presented.

It is concluded that (1) the differences between adult and childhood non-Hodgkin's lymphoma in presentation and response to therapy can be accounted for by the relative frequencies of the different phenotypically-defined subclasses in these age groups; and (2) future studies of childhood non-Hodgkin's lymphoma should take account of the phenotypic variants of histologically defined subclasses of this disease.

ACKNOWLEDGMENTS

The author would like to acknowledge the co-operation of the Chairman, Dr. John Martin, and members of the United Kingdom Children's Cancer Study Group for the availability of biopsy material from their patients. He would also like to thank Dr. A. G. Stansfeld of St. Bartholomew's Hospital, London, for his histological review of the cases.

References

1. Gerard-Marchant R, Hamblin I, Lennert K, *et al*: Classification of non-Hodgkin's lymphomas. *Lancet 2:406–408, 1974.*
2. Greaves MF, Janossy G: Patterns of gene expression and the cellular origins of human leukaemias. *Biochim Biophys Acta 516:193–230, 1978.*
3. Greaves MF: Membrane antigens and enzymatic phenotypes in leukaemia; correlates of normal haemopoetic differentiation? In Serrou B, Rosenfeld C (eds): *Human Lymphocyte Differentiation: Its Application to Cancer.* Elsevier/North-Holland Biomedical Press, New York, 1978, pp. 253–264.
4. Vogler LB, Crist WM, Cooper MD, Lawton AR: Acute lymphocytic leukaemia involving pre-B cells, in Serrou B, Rosenfeld C (eds): *Human Lymphocyte Differentiation: Its Application to Cancer.* Elsevier/North-Holland Biomedical Press, New York, 1978, pp. 407–413.
5. Touraine JL: A model of sequential differentiation and ontogeny of T lymphocytes in man, in Serrou B, Rosenfeld C (eds): *Human Lymphocyte Differentiation: Its Application to Cancer.* Elsevier/North-Holland Biomedical Press, New York, 1978, pp. 93–100.
6. Sigal NH, Klinman NR: The B-cell clonotype repertoire. Adv Immunol 26:255—337, 1978.
7. Janossy G, Goldstone AHM, Capellaro D, *et al*: Differentiation-linked expression of p 28 33 (Ia-like) structures on human leukaemic cells. *Br J Haematol 37:391–402, 1977.*
8. Humphreys RE, McCune JMM, Chess L, *et al*: Isolation and immunological characterisation of a human B lymphocyte specific, cell surface antigen. *J Exp Med 144:98, 1976.*
9. Bollum FJ: Terminal deoxynucleotidyl transferase, in Boyer PD (ed): *The Enzymes* (edn. 3). Academic, New York, 1974, pp. 145–171.
10. McCaffrey R, Harrison TA, Parkman R, Baltimore D: Terminal deoxynucleotidyl transferase activity in human leukaemic cells and immature thymocytes. *N Engl J Med 292:775, 1975.*
11. Gregoire KE, Goldschneider I, Barton RW, Bollum FJ: Intracellular distribution of terminal deoxynucleotidyl transferase in rat bone marrow and thymus. *Proc Natl Acad Sci 74:3993, 1977.*
12. Kung PC, Long JC, McCaffrey KP, *et al*: Terminal deoxynucleotidyl transferase in the diagnosis of leukaemia and lymphoma. *Am. J Med 64:788–789, 1978.*
13. Moretta L, Webb SR, Grossi CE, *et al*: Functional analysis of two human T-cell subpopulations. Help and suppression of B-cell responses by T cells bearing receptors for IgM or IgG. *J Exp Med 146:184–200, 1977.*
14. Herberman RB, DJeu JY, Kay HD, *et al*: Natural killer cells; characteristics and regulation of activity. *Immunol Rev 44:43–70, 1979.*
15. Fridman WH, Yagello M, Rabourdin C, Gisler RH: T cell Fc receptor and its role in the differentiation of T and B cells, in Serrou B, Rosenfeld C (eds): *Human Lymphocyte Differentiation, Its Application to Cancer.* Elsevier/North-Holland Biomedical Press, New York, 1978, pp. 51–60.
16. Stein H, Siemssen U, Lennert K: Complement receptor subtypes C3b and C3d in lymphatic tissue and follicular lymphomas. *Br J Cancer 37:520–529, 1978.*

17. Greaves MF, Janossy G, Roberts M, *et al*: Membrane phenotyping, diagnosis, monitoring and classification of acute "lymphoid" leukaemias. *Haematol Bluttransfus 20:61–75, 1977.*
18. Niaudet P, Greaves MF: Identification of T lineage associated membrane proteins, in Serrou B, Rosenfeld C (eds): *Human Lymphocyte Differentiation; Its Application to Cancer.* Elsevier/North-Holland Biomedical Press, New York, 1978, pp. 117–121.
19. Dickler HB, Adkinson NF, Terry WD: Evidence for individual human peripheral blood lymphocytes bearing both B and T cell markers. *Nature (New Biol) 247:213–215, 1974.*
20. Chiao JW, Pantic VS, Good RA: Human peripheral blood lymphocytes bearing both B cell complement receptors and T cell characteristics for sheep erythrocytes detected by a mixed rosette method. *Clin Exp Immunol 18:483–490, 1974.*
21. Moretta L, Mingari MC, Moretta A, Lydyard PM: Receptors for IgM are expressed on acute lymphoblastic leukaemic cells having T cell characteristics. *Clin Immunol Immunopathol 7:405–409, 1977.*
22. Stein H, Petersen N, Gaedicke G, *et al*: Lymphoblastic leukaemia of convoluted or acid phosphatase positive type, a tumour of T precursor cells. *Int J Cancer 17:292–295, 1976.*
23. Pilcher WJ, Lum L, Broder S: Fc receptors on human T lymphocytes. I. Transition of Tγ to Tμ cells. *J Immunol 121:1540–1548, 1978.*
24. Pearl ER, Vogler LB, Okos AJ, *et al*: B lymphocyte precursors in human bone marrow: an analysis of normal individuals and patients with antibody deficiency states. *J Immunol 120:1169–1174, 1978.*
25. Vogler LB, Crist WM, Bockman DE, *et al*: Pre-B cell leukaemia; a new phenotype of childhood lymphoblastic leukaemia. *N Engl J Med 298:872–878, 1978.*
26. Kearney JF, Cooper MD, Lawton AR: B lymphocyte differentiation induced by lipopolysaccharide. III. Suppression of B cell maturation by anti-mouse immunoglobulin antibodies. *J Immunol 16:1664–1668, 1976.*
27. Abbot J, Hoffmann MK, Chen AF, Hammerling U: Sequential appearance of surface markers in the ontogeny of B lymphocytes, in Muller Berart N, Rosenfeld C, Tarin D, Visa D (eds): *Progress in Differentiation Research.* Elsevier/North-Holland Biomedical Press, New York, 1976, pp. 545–550.
28. Embling PH, Evans H, Guttierez C, *et al*: The structural requirements for immunoglobulin aggregates to localize in germinal centres. *Immunology 34:781, 1978.*
29. White RG, Henderson DC, Eslami MB, Nielsen KH: Localization of protein antigen in the chicken spleen; effect of various manipulative procedure on the morphogenesis of the germinal centre. *Immunology 28:1, 1975.*
30. Nieuwenhuis P, Van-Nouhuijs CE, Eggens JH, Keuning, FJ: Germinal centres and the origin of the B-cell system. I. Germinal centres in the rabbit appendix. *Immunology 26:497–507, 1974.*
31. Nieuwenhuis P, Keuning FJ: Germinal centres and the origin of the B-cell system. II. Germinal centres in the rabbit spleen and popliteal lymph nodes. *Immunology 26:509, 1974.*
32. Insel RA, Merler E: The necessity for T cell help for human tonsil B cell responses to pokeweek mitogen; induction of DNA synthesis, immunoglobulin and specific antibody production with a T helper factor produced with pokeweed mitogen. *J Immunol 118:2009, 1977.*
33. Davies AJS, Carter RL, Leuchars E, *et al*: The morphology of immune reactions in normal, thymectomised and reconstituted mice. I. The response to sheep erythrocytes. *Immunology 16:57–59, 1969.*
34. Coccia PF: Characterization of the blast cell in childhood non-Hodgkin's lymphoproliferative malignancies. *Semin Oncol 4:287–296, 1977.*
35. Hammerling J, Chen AF, Abbott J: The ontogeny of murine B lymphocytes II. The sequence of B cell differentiation from surface Ig negative precursors to plasma cells. *Proc Natl Acad Sci USA 73:2008, 1976.*
36. Harris NS: Plasma cell surface antigen on human blood lymphocytes. *Nature 250:507–509, 1974.*

37. Gathings WE, Lawton AR, Cooper MD: Immunofluorescent studies of the development of the pre B cells, B lymphocytes, and immunoglobulin isotype diversity in humans. *Eur J Immunol 7:804, 1977.*
38. Seligmann M, Preud'Homme JL, Brouet JC: B and T cell markers in human proliferative blood diseases and primary immunodeficiencies with special reference to membrane bound immunoglobulin. *Transplant Rev 16:85–113, 1973.*
39. Lennert K: *Lymphomas Other than Hodgkin's Disease.* Springer-Verlag, New York, 1978.
40. Rappaport H: *Tumours of the Haematopoietic System. Atlas of Tumour Pathology,* Section 3. Armed Forces Institute of Pathology, Washington, D.C., 1966.
41. Greaves MF: Personal communication to the author, 1979.
42. Habeshaw, J, Catley P, Stansfeld A, Brearley R: Surface phenotype, histology, and the nature of non-Hodgkin's lymphoma. *Br J Cancer, 1979* (in press).
43. Williams AH, Taylor CR, Higgins GR, *et al*: Childhood lymphoma-leukemia. I. Correlation of morphology and immunological studies. *Cancer 42:171–181, 1978.*
44. Berard CW, Jaffe ES, Braylan RC, *et al*: Immunological aspects and pathology of the malignant lymphomas. *Cancer 42:911–921, 1978.*
45. Coccia PF, Kersey JH, Gajl-Peczalska KJ, *et al*: Prognostic significance of surface marker analysis in childhood non-Hodgkin lymphoproliferative malignancies. *Am J Hematol 1:405–417, 1976.*
46. Brunning RD, McKenna RW, Bloomfield CD, *et al*: Bone marrow involvement in Burkitt's lymphoma. *Cancer 40:1771–1779, 1977.*
47. Donlon JA, Jaffe ES, Braylan RC: Terminal deoxynucleotidyl transferase activity in malignant lymphomas. *N Engl J Med 297:461–464, 1977.*
48. Kung PC, Long JC, McCaffrey RP, *et al*: Terminal deoxynucleotidyl transferase in the diagnosis of leukaemia and lymphoma. *Am J Med 64:788–797, 1978.*
49. Kersey JH, Gajl-Peczalska KJ, Coccia PF, Nesbit ME: The nature of childhood leukaemia and lymphoma. *Am J Pathol 90:487–496, 1978.*
50. Barrett SG, Schwade JG, Ranken R, Kadin MD: Lymphoblasts with both B and T markers in childhood leukaemia and lymphoma. *Blood 50:71–79, 1977.*
51. Bardosi L, Nemeth P, Kelnyi G: Double labelled cells in a malignant lymphoma (thymoma) (Letter). *Br J Haematol 37:151–152, 1977.*
52. Dehner LP: Non-Hodgkin's lymphomas and malignant histiocytosis in children. *Semin Oncol 4:273–286, 1977.*
53. Robinowitz BN, Noguchi S, Bergfeld WF: Tumour cell characterisation of histiocytic medullary reticulosis. *Arch Dermatol 113:927–929, 1977.*

CHAPTER FOUR

Diagnosis and Staging of Non-Hodgkin's Lymphoma in Childhood

STUART R. TOLEDANO, MD; ANNA T. MEADOWS, MD

THE HETEROGENEITY OF THE group of diseases known collectively as the malignant non-Hodgkin's lymphomas (NHL) is especially apparent in children. These tumors arise from cells of the lymphoreticular system, and the malignant cells can demonstrate the full range of behavior found in their benign counterparts. While the lack of uniformity of both pathologic and clinical manifestations can confuse the physician, this same variability has enabled basic scientists to uncover clues to the functional ontogeny of the immune system. Thus, an understanding of the biologic characteristics of lymphoid cells in various stages of differentiation may be expected to emerge from the study of these tumors.

In this chapter, we will try to classify these "mistakes of nature" in ways that are physiologically rational and therapeutically useful. Diagnosis and staging will be considered with particular reference to a classification scheme that is both functionally and clinically relevant.

EPIDEMIOLOGY

In western nations, non-Hodgkin's lymphomas comprise about 10% of pediatric cancers. These tumors occur at a frequency similar to the common embryonal tumors, Wilms' tumor and neuroblastoma, that is, seven to eight per million per year from birth to 15 years.[1] However, a relatively high incidence of non-Hodgkin's lymphoma, Burkitt's type, has been observed in parts of Africa. This has been attributed to factors of climate that foster a high prevalence of malaria.[2,3] Unlike acute lymphocytic leukemia (ALL), these diseases are more prevalent in the school-age child than in the preschooler. Unlike Hodgkin's disease, the

Division of Oncology, The Children's Hospital of Philadelphia, 34th Street and Civic Center Blvd., Philadelphia, PA 19104

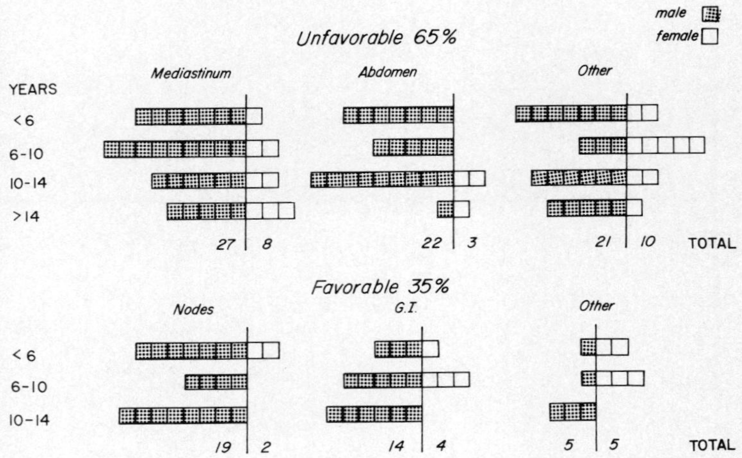

FIG. 1. Distribution of 140 patients with non-Hodgkin's lymphoma entered in the Children's Cancer Study Group, protocol 551, with classification according to site, age, sex, and extent of disease.

non-Hodgkin's lymphomas do not show a rising incidence throughout childhood.[4] Like Hodgkin's disease, however, there is a preference for males over females. The age and sex distribution of 140 consecutively registered new patients in the Children's Cancer Study Group (CCSG) protocol 551 demonstrates these demographic characteristics (Fig. 1). It can also be seen from this figure that 65% of the children have the "unfavorable" type, that is, the type that is unresectable or involves sites that have had a poor response to therapy in the past, such as the mediastinum, bone marrow, or CNS.[5]

Children with immunodeficiency diseases are at special risk for developing non-Hodgkin's lymphomas. Like the athymic (nude) mouse, they are not predisposed in general to cancer, but acquire NHL at a rate which exceeds that of the normal child by 100 times.[6] Renal transplant recipients have an excess of lymphoma, especially reticulum cell sarcoma of the brain.[7] It has been suggested that the suppression of the immune system necessary for the preservation of the graft, and the presence of a constant antigenic stimulus, are responsible for this excess incidence of lymphomas.

DIAGNOSIS

The sites of involvement and hence the clinical manifestations of childhood non-Hodgkin's lymphomas are diverse. These tumors arise wherever lymphoid tissue is found. They often appear in a characteristic way, and the diagnosis may be obvious from the clinical presentation. Common sites include peripheral lymph nodes, Peyer's patches in the intestines, thymus gland, and Waldeyer's ring. Less often, non-Hodgkin's lymphomas arise in the breast, central nervous system, kidney, liver, lung or pleura, nasopharynx, orbit, ovary, parotid gland, prostate, skin, spleen, stomach, testes, and thyroid. Involvement may be limited initially to a single site of origin, but more often in childhood, the lymphoma is advanced in stage and a single primary site may not be apparent. Since there is a propensity for early marrow involvement, it is often difficult to distinguish acute lymphocytic leukemia from a small primary lymphoma with early bone marrow involvement.

There are, however, certain clinical features that have been noted in distinguishing NHL in bone marrow from acute lymphocytic leukemia. In NHL, the peripheral blood count may be normal or nearly so, with hemoglobin concentration no less than 9.0 g/dl and platelet count no less than 100,000/mm^3. No circulating immature cells are seen, and the differential leukocyte count may show adequate numbers of granulocytes. Some investigators assign an arbitrary number of lymphoblasts in marrow as a criterion for the diagnosis of non-Hodgkin's lymphoma, such as less than 25%. We have seen individuals, however, with isolated lymphomas of bone and skin, with as many as 70% of the nucleated marrow cells being lymphoblasts, and a clinical presentation unlike acute lymphocytic leukemia. These patients are probably more like those with non-Hodgkin's lymphoma as to responsiveness to therapy, ultimate outcome, and the biological nature of the malignant cell. The distinction between these clinical entities may be less apparent if one considers functional characteristics of the malignant cell or response to chemotherapy in making a diagnosis. Thus, "T" cell non-Hodgkin's lymphoma is as resistant to attempts at cure as "T" cell acute leukemia.

Initial evaluation includes a careful history and physical examination. Specific inquiry should be made regarding the ingestion of diphenylhydantoin and trauma from cat scratches, both of which can cause benign lymphadenopathy. Histologic examination of malignant cells is crucial to the diagnosis. These may be obtained from tissue, such as that obtained by excisional or other biopsies, or from effusions, such as pleural or pericardial fluid or ascites. Often, there is no opportunity to select the appropriate tissue, since the presentation is acute, as is the case with abdominal or mediastinal disease. However, a node for biopsy should be carefully selected since its architectural pattern can be contributory to the diagnosis. Cells should be subject to examination for surface markers that distinguish between the subtypes of lymphoblasts; such surface marker studies may help determine the therapeutic approach and also offer prognostic clues. These characteristics are discussed in detail elsewhere in this book (see Chapter 3).

A minimum diagnostic workup in any child with non-Hodgkin's lymphoma includes the following studies (Table 1): a complete blood count, including a differential leukocyte count, platelet count, and examination of the peripheral smear with attention to any atypical cells; urinalysis, with attention to the presence of red cells, protein and uric acid crystals; a chemical screening profile, especially

TABLE 1
Diagnostic and Staging Studies for Childhood Non-Hodgkin's Lymphoma

Minimum studies	Optional studies
1. Examination of malignant cells by histopathology and surface markers	1. Skeletal survey and bone scan
2. Complete blood count with differential leukocyte and platelet counts	2. Barium studies of the intestinal tract
3. Urinalysis	3. Intravenous pyelography
4. Serum uric acid, blood urea nitrogen, serum creatinine, SGOT, SGPT, serum bilirubin	4. Chest tomography
5. Chest roentgenogram	5. Liver-spleen scan
6. Bone marrow aspirates from multiple sites	6. Gallium scan
7. Cerebrospinal fluid cell count, cytology, glucose and protein	7. Ultrasonography
	8. Computerized axial tomography

tests measuring serum uric acid, liver function, and kidney function; chest roentgenogram; bone marrow aspirate, preferably from at least two sites; and cerebrospinal fluid examination. The CSF examination should include glucose, protein, white cell number, and examination of any cells on a cytocentrifuged or millipore filter preparation. Bone marrow biopsies, which have been found to be more useful than aspirates in adults, have been recommended for children with lymphomas.[8] However, the superiority of the bone marrow biopsy over the aspiration technique has not been demonstrated in children.[9] Multiple aspirates are suggested, since in about 10% of patients clusters of abnormal cells may be present in only one site of the several sites sampled.[10]

An initial skeletal survey is useful, especially if localized bone pain or swelling is present. A radionuclide bone scan would be a more sensitive indicator of bony involvement and, at the same time, may yield useful information pertaining to renal function. Contrast studies of the bowel should be performed if intraabdominal pathology is suspected. The barium studies, however, may fail to reveal abnormalities, and intraabdominal disease may be found at laparotomy.[11] Ultrasonography may aid in the definition and identification of intraabdominal masses. Intravenous pyelography, often suggested as part of the initial workup, may reveal enlarged retroperitoneal lymph nodes or lymphomatous kidney involvement. Conventional tomography has proven useful in defining the extent of disease in the nasopharynx, paranasal sinuses, and mediastinum.[12] Radionuclide studies are often recommended, but the results of liver-spleen scans are often equivocal,[11,12] and gallium scans, which are most accurate in the thorax, where conventional radiographic studies provide adequate information, are unreliable in defining intraabdominal disease.[13]

Computerized axial tomography is a sensitive noninvasive method of detecting the presence of tumor and defining its extent within the head and neck as well as within the abdomen. However, the usefulness of computerized tomography may be reduced in children since they have less visceral fat with which organs and masses may be outlined.[14] Lymphangiography and staging laparotomy are generally not performed in children who present with extraabdominal lymphomas.[11,12] Only rarely would the results of lymphangiography and staging laparotomy affect the plan of therapy; on the other hand, lymphangiography may actually be contraindicated in patients with respiratory impairment because of the risk of lipid pneumonitis. Also, laparotomy would significantly delay treatment of a disease known for early dissemination.

STAGING

A stage is assigned prior to initiation of therapy and following diagnosis and evaluation of extent of disease. An adequate staging system that is easy to remember and simple to apply should have four characteristics[11,15]: it should (1) be based upon the natural history of the disease and the biologic behavior of the tumor, (2) assist the oncologist in the selection of the most appropriate therapeutic modalities available, (3) provide prognostic information based upon the site and extent of disease, and (4) permit the comparison of therapeutic results between various institutions when a standardized system is used.

Currently, however, there is concern regarding the applicability to non-Hodgkin's lymphomas in children of the staging system in widespread use for lymphomas, namely, the staging system developed in Ann Arbor in 1970.[16] This staging system was developed and has been useful for Hodgkin's disease in children and adults but its usefulness even in adult non-Hodgkin's lymphomas is now being questioned.[15] In Table 2 the Ann Arbor system is compared with two recently developed staging schemas.[9,17] These alternative staging systems consider the unique characteristics of non-Hodgkin's lymphomas in children as well as the deficiencies of the Ann Arbor classification.[11,18] These special considerations include the following: (1) the noncontiguous spread of the disease in children with its propensity for leukemic conversion and CNS involvement; (2) the fact that disease localized to the mediastinum (Ann Arbor stage I) may carry a particularly poor prognosis; (3) the rarity of true Ann Arbor stage III patients; and (4) the questionable value of rigorous pathologic staging with an exploratory laparotomy in a disease characterized by early widespread dissemination, and the questionable value of splenectomy with the known risk of overwhelming sepsis.

The St. Jude system is precise enough so that the results of different therapies can be compared.[9] No distinction is made by investigators at the Memorial

TABLE 2
Comparison of Staging Schema for Childhood Non-Hodgkin's Lymphoma

	Ann Arbor[16]	St. Jude Children's Research Hospital[9]	Memorial Sloan-Kettering Cancer Center[17]
Stage I	Involvement of a single lymph node region (I) or of a single extra-lymphatic organ or site (I_E).	A single tumor (extranodal) or single anatomic area (nodal), with the exclusion of mediastinum or abdomen.	One single site.
Stage II	Involvement of two or more lymphoid regions on the same side of the diaphragm (II) or localized involvement of extra-lymphatic organ or site and of one or more lymph node regions on the same side of the diaphragm (II_E).	A single tumor (extranodal) with regional node involvement. Two or more nodal areas on the same side of the diaphragm. Two single (extranodal) tumors with or without regional node involvement on the same side of the diaphragm. A primary GI tract tumor, usually in the ileocecal area, with or without involvement of associated mesenteric nodes only.	Two or more sites above or below the diaphragm.
Stage III	Involvement of lymph node regions on both side of the diaphragm (III), which may also be accompanied by localized involvement of extra-lymphatic organ or site (III_E) or by splenic involvement (III_S) or both III_{SE}).	Two single tumors (extranodal) on opposite sides of the diaphragm. Two or more nodal areas above and below the diaphragm. All the primary intrathoracic tumors (mediastinal, pleural, thymic). All extensive primary intraabdominal disease.	Two or more sites above and below the diaphragm. Extensive intra-thoracic. Extensive intraabdominal.
Stage IV	Diffuse or disseminated involvement of one or more extralymphatic organs or tissues with or without associated lymph node enlargement.	Any of the above with initial CNS and/or bone marrow involvement.	One of the above with bone marrow and/or central nervous system involvement.

Sloan-Kettering Cancer Center between leukemia (more than 25% abnormal cells in the bone marrow or the presence of circulating blasts) and lymphoma with bone marrow involvement.[10] Most investigators distinguish between acute lymphocytic leukemia with involvement of the spleen and lymph nodes on the one hand and lymphoma on the other. Still another classification scheme is that tentatively used by the Children's Cancer Study Group.[5] Localized and resectable lymphoma, with or without adjacent lymph node involvement, is called "favorable"; while lymphoma with mediastinal, diffuse abdominal, osseous, or nervous system involvement is called "unfavorable." Bone marrow involvement is "unfavorable" and is defined as presence of greater than 5% but fewer than 25% abnormal cells in an aspirate. This system has the advantage of combining simplicity with relevance and may provide consistency in predicting outcome for children. Further refinement of the staging of non-Hodgkin's lymphomas in children will result when information regarding site and extent of disease is combined with histopathology and immunopathology of these tumors.

ABDOMINAL NON-HODGKIN'S LYMPHOMA

The abdomen is the most common site of origin of non-Hodgkin's lymphoma in children and accounts for up to 45% of reported cases.[19] Overall, one-half have lymphoma limited to a segment of bowel, with or without mesenteric lymph node involvement. The remainder have extensive disease with retroperitoneal or paraaortic lymph node involvement, seeding of the mesentery or peritoneum, or direct infiltration of structures adjacent to the primary tumor. In the Children's Cancer Study Group lymphoma study, 60% of children with abdominal non-Hodgkin's lymphoma had widespread disease (Fig. 1). Certain centers, because of particular referral patterns, report more or less localized involvement. For example, in the Memorial Sloan-Kettering Cancer Center series, 76% of the abdominal tumors were unresectable[20] and in the St. Jude series, 68% were unresectable.[21]

Burkitt's lymphoma is a type of diffuse undifferentiated lymphocytic lymphoma originally reported as a jaw tumor in East African children.[22] Tumors that are clinically and pathologically similar have been reported in North American children, but with some differences. In the American patients, there is a greater frequency of abdominal involvement and leukemic transformation than in the African form, and the Epstein-Barr virus genome is rarely present.[23]

Abdominal non-Hodgkin's lymphoma is primarily a disease of school-aged boys. In Jenkin's series the male/female ratio was 9:1;[19] it was 10:1 in the Denver report,[24] and 5:1 in the Children's Cancer Study Group report (Fig. 1). Abdominal lymphomas are rare before the age of 2 years, and children over 10 years appear to have a more unfavorable prognosis.

Pain is the most common complaint of a child with an abdominal lymphoma. The pain may be referred to the chest, shoulders, legs, or back if the primary is not within the bowel. Other signs and symptoms include vomiting and diarrhea, fever, abdominal distension, anorexia, weight loss, gastrointestinal bleeding, ascites, paraplegia, and menstrual irregularities. Although Jenkin reports that in a majority of the children a mass was palpable,[19] others have found this sign to be less frequent.[20]

A child with widespread abdominal lymphoma presents with a history of a rapidly enlarging abdomen over a short period of time. Often examination will reveal fluid in addition to the presence of a mass. This, together with an elevated serum uric acid, is characteristic of the undifferentiated, pleomorphic or Burkitt's type of lymphoma. Characteristic lymphoblasts may be seen in cytocentrifuged preparations of ascitic fluid. Surface marker studies may be performed on these cells. These cases do not pose a diagnostic problem, but require careful pretreatment attention to fluid and electrolyte balance and assessment of renal function.

An unusual presentation recently encountered by the authors involved a 13-year-old boy, who had several weeks of abdominal pain that culminated in acute pancreatitis. This latter diagnosis was based on an elevated serum amylase level, but there was no history of trauma or infection and no underlying hematologic abnormalities. When it was appreciated that his abdomen was enlarging with accumulation of fluid and the presence of a mass, a peritoneal tap was performed. The diagnosis of B-cell non-Hodgkin's lymphoma was made on the basis of the morphologic surface marker characteristics of the malignant cells examined.

Another typical clinical presentation is that of the preschooler or school-age child who presents with an acute abdomen. Possible preoperative diagnoses include appendicitis, ruptured viscus, and intestinal obstruction. An intestinal lymphoma may also be the lead point of an intussusception. The diagnosis of lymphoma is often made at laparotomy by biopsy of lymphoid tissue if the lymphoma is widespread or by resection of a segment of intestine if the lymphoma is localized. Tissue processed for surface markers can be helpful in determining the characteristics and origin of the malignant cells.

Although the prognosis for a child with an abdominal non-Hodgkin's lymphoma is dependent on the tumor bulk and its extent of resectability,[9] a formal staging laparotomy is neither recommended nor indicated. This assertion is made because the clinical findings and the presence of bone marrow or CNS involvement provide the best prognostic criteria.[18] A cure rate of greater than 70% can be expected in a case of a localized gastrointestinal tumor after complete gross resection and whole abdominal irradiation.[19,20,25] Recommendations for optimal therapy of extensive intraabdominal lymphoma have included removal of tumor bulk if technically possible,[26] and the administration of a program of multiagent chemotherapy.[9] Although radiation therapy and second-look surgery for nonresectable lymphoma have been recommended,[10,27] data supporting an advantage for these strategies is lacking.

The risk of leukemic transformation is less when the primary tumor is intraabdominal than when it is in the mediastinum or in peripheral lymph nodes.[9,11,24,27] However, it is not rare to see bone marrow involvement at the time of diagnosis in a child with extensive intraabdominal disease; in this group the risk of leukemic conversion is between 10% and 23%.[11,24,25,28,29] The 20% incidence of CNS involvement after leukemic conversion in these patients may be an underestimate since lumbar punctures are not routinely performed.[25] While the bone marrow may be the site of first relapse, the CNS has never been reported as the initial site of relapse after complete resection of a localized gastrointestinal tumor.[24,25,27]

Critical problems with nomenclature and classification make it difficult to determine the relationship between histology, site and extent of disease, and outcome. In the three series, which included 46 patients, utilizing the Rappaport classification,[30] poorly differentiated lymphocytic lymphoma occurred with the greatest frequency (54%).[11,20,24] Employing the morphologic criteria devised by Lukes *et al.*,[31] two other series found the majority of abdominal lymphomas (21 out of 37) to be of the small noncleaved follicular center cell type.[25,32] Cells from abdominal lymphomas that have been examined express monoclonal immunoglobulin (which is a B-cell characteristic) but do not form spontaneous rosettes with sheep erythrocytes (which is a T-cell characteristic).[32] More precise and standardized descriptions of the malignant cells may make it possible to correlate outcome following a specific therapy with histologic and functional characteristics.

An illustrative case. A 13-year-old black boy presented with a three-week history of increasing fatigue, malaise, fever, night sweats, anorexia, abdominal pain, and a 17-lb weight loss.

One week prior to admission, a mass developed on the left side of the neck and he was treated with cephalexin without improvement. Positive physical findings included a 3.5 × 3.0-cm lymph node at the angle of the jaw on the left. Palpation of the abdomen revealed a liver edge 2.0 cm below the right costal margin, a palpable spleen tip, and the presence of a 5 × 6-cm right upper quadrant mass and 3 × 2-cm right lower quadrant mass. Laboratory data were as follows: hemoglobin 11.1 g/dl; platelet count 60,000/mm^3; white blood cell count 5,300/mm^3, with a differential count showing 35% polymorphonuclear leukocytes, 5% bands, 4% eosinophils, 4% monocytes, and 53% lymphocytes, several of which were blastlike in appearance; the blood urea nitrogen level 16 mg/dl; serum creatinine 1.2 mg/dl; and serum uric acid 15.6 mg/dl. The chest film showed mediastinal widening with marked hilar adenopathy. An upper gastrointestinal series with small bowel follow-through demonstrated intrinsic masses in the stomach, duodenum, and distal ileum (Fig. 2A). An intravenous pyelogram showed poor visualization and enlargement of the lower pole of the left kidney (Fig. 2B). A bone marrow aspirate revealed that 91% of the cells were large, vacuolated lymphoblasts. Surface immunoglobulin M was found on 55% of these cells, and 45% of the cells ingested latex particles.

After fluid balance and a normal serum uric acid level were achieved with vigorous hydration and administration of allopurinol, chemotherapy was begun with cyclophosphamide, vincristine, prednisone, intravenous

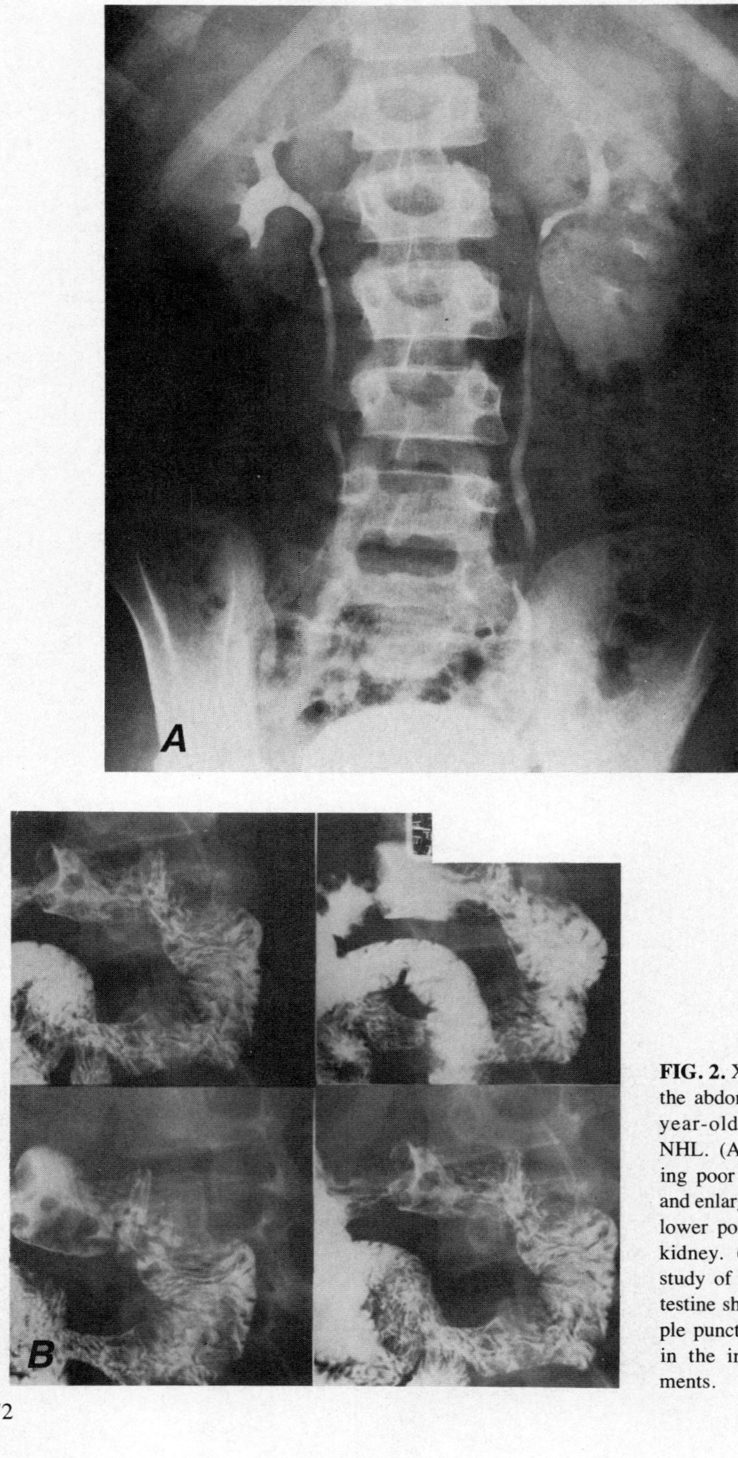

FIG. 2. X-ray films of the abdomen of a 13-year-old boy with NHL. (A) IVP showing poor visualization and enlargement of the lower pole of the left kidney. (B) Contrast study of the small intestine showing multiple punctate lucencies in the involved segments.

methotrexate and intrathecal methotrexate. A complete remission was achieved within six weeks.

This was a case of non-Hodgkin's lymphoma with intraabdominal primary tumor and with early leukemic transformation. There was rapid and dramatic response to a program of intensive multidrug chemotherapy.

MEDIASTINAL NON-HODGKIN'S LYMPHOMA

The epidemiologic, clinical, and cellular characteristics of mediastinal non-Hodgkin's lymphoma and of acute lymphocytic leukemia with an anterior mediastinal mass are so similar as to make separation of these two entities quite difficult and often aribtrary. Indeed, diffuse undifferentiated or lymphoblastic non-Hodgkin's lymphoma cannot be separated from acute leukemia by morphologic or cytologic criteria.[33] Both show a male predominance, a similar age range, an aggressive clinical course characterized by early involvement of the meninges and testes, and similar cellular characteristics. The rate of transformation of a mediastinal non-Hodgkin's lymphoma to leukemia is extremely rapid[11,28]; and when this occurs, it is almost uniformly fatal.[10,24,33]

The mediastinum is the primary site of non-Hodgkin's lymphoma in 15–45% of patients.[10,11,24,29,34] Of the 166 children with non-Hodgkin's lymphomas enrolled in the Children's Cancer Study Group protocol 551 study, 39 (23%) had mediastinal tumors. The male-to-female sex ratio varies from 1:1 to 3:1,[10,11,24] and the children are of school age. Since the outlook for these patients has been dismal, most staging systems place children with anterior mediastinal masses in an advanced stage, usually stage III.[9,17] If bone marrow or CNS involvement is also present, they fall into stage IV.

Dyspnea, cough, and wheeze are frequent symptoms. Often, these symptoms are acute, and the patient is in extreme respiratory distress when first seen. Fever, fatigue, anorexia, nausea, weight loss, peripheral lymphadenopathy, and substernal, pleuritic, or abdominal pain are less common. The superior vena cava syndrome may be present and may mimic angioneurotic edema. The occurrence of this syndrome accompanied by wheezing may be interpreted as "allergy or asthma" by the physician. Pleural effusions are common and, rarely, pericardial effusion with tamponade may be the presenting symptom.

The histopathology of the mediastinal tumor is most often established by biopsy of the intrathoracic mass. However, in a large proportion of cases, the diagnosis may be made from biopsy of a cervical or scalene lymph node, from biopsy of chest wall extension of the tumor, or from the finding of malignant lymphoma cells in pleural or pericardial fluid. These methods of obtaining diagnostic material are encouraged, since children with mediastinal non-Hodgkin's lymphoma may be poor risks for anesthesia because of their compromised respiratory status. On occasion, a presumptive diagnosis of non-Hodgkin's lymphoma will be established when a child with an anterior mediastinal mass and marked respiratory embarrassment, too ill to undergo general anesthesia and a thoracotomy, is empirically started on corticosteroids. Although surgery may be scheduled several days after the commencement of corticosteroid therapy, there is often dramatic and complete resolution of the mediastinal mass, and the tissue obtained is interpreted as "necrotic thymus." This characteristic clinical presentation, the demonstration on a lateral chest film of a mass in the anterior mediastinum, and the prompt response to corticosteroid therapy provide strong presumptive evidence for the diagnosis of mediastinal non-Hodgkin's lymphoma.

Although a precise and widely accepted histopathologic classification of mediastinal lymphomas is not yet available, it appears that these tumors arise from the thymus gland. Studies using the Rappaport classification[16] show that nodular lymphomas rarely occur in the mediastinum and indicate that this classification scheme is probably not applicable to lymphomas occurring in children. The majority of mediastinal lymphomas in children are classified as diffuse, poorly differentiated lymphocytic or undifferentiated lymphocytic.[11,24,33,35] The term malignant lymphoma, lymphoblastic type has been applied to a subset of diffuse poorly differentiated lymphocytic lymphomas that are characterized by a high mitotic index and such immaturity of the lymphoid cells as to make them indistinguishable from the lymphoblasts and prolymphocytes of acute lymphocytic leukemia.[36] Clinical characteristics of this subset include frequent occurrence in older children and adolescents, the presence of mediastinal masses in 50% of cases, and a rapidly progressive course with subsequent bone marrow and central nervous system involvement. In 50% of patients with lymphoblastic lymphoma and a mediastinal mass, nuclear convolutions are recognized.

When classified according to the scheme of Lukes and Collins,[31] a high positive correlation exists among the presence of nuclear convolutions, a mediastinal mass, and the percent of E-rosette-forming cells, the latter being a T-cell characteristic.[32] This distinctive morphology is not observed in patients with small noncleaved lymphoma/leukemia, nor in those patients with acute lymphocytic leukemia whose cells do not form E-rosettes. Other investigators have confirmed the association between the presence of a mediastinal mass, the finding of lymphoblastic cells or convoluted cell lymphoma, and the probable thymic origin of this tumor as suggested by the frequency of rosette formation.[37-40] These cells are also positive for the enzymatic marker terminal deoxynucleotidyl transferase (TdT), and they possess human T-lymphocyte antigens,[18,41] features that are also found in cases of acute lymphocytic leukemia accompanied by a mediastinal mass.

Since more than 80% of children with mediastinal non-Hodgkin's lymphoma develop acute leukemia, usually within the first year, the distinction between NHL and ALL at the time of diagnosis may be arbitrary. Some oncologists treat children with a mediastinal mass and with greater than 25% blast forms in the bone marrow the same as patients with acute lymphocytic leukemia. On the other hand, others treat ALL with anterior mediastinal masses the same as NHL, regardless of the percentage of leukemic cells in the bone marrow. It behooves investigators reporting the results of clinical trials to distinguish between anterior mediastinal masses and hilar lymphadenopathy, since hilar adenopathy may reflect generalized nodal involvement in a child with null cell or the common form of acute lymphocytic leukemia. The latter child has a more favorable outlook, and the results of treatment are not comparable to those obtained in cases of true mediastinal non-Hodgkin's lymphoma.

In recent years, it has become apparent that aggressive chemotherapy may prevent leukemic conversion, and indeed, the survival of patients with mediastinal non-Hodgkin's lymphoma has improved. Prior to 1973, there were no long-term survivors among 11 children with mediastinal NHL treated at the M.D. Anderson Hospital[28] and no two-year survivors among 10 children treated at the Memorial Sloan-Kettering Cancer Center.[10] Improved results have been obtained at the latter institution and by other investigators using multiple agent chemotherapy.[11,41,42] Although 7 of the 19 mediastinal NHL patients in the Memorial Sloan-Kettering Cancer Center series had bone marrow involvement at diagnosis, actuarial survival for this group was 88% at two years; at the time of that report 50% of these children were off therapy. Modifications of this LSA2-L2 protocol and of other chemotherapy protocols are now undergoing clinical trials. The results of these trials are expected to change the outlook for children with malignant mediastinal lymphomas.

An illustrative case. A two-year-old black girl was admitted to the Children's Hospital of Philadelphia because of increasing irritability and intermittent cyanosis due to respiratory distress. She was being treated with penicillin for pneumonitis that had been confirmed radiographically two weeks earlier. Although the fever defervesced, a wet cough persisted. When the chest film was repeated, an anterior mediastinal mass, marked tracheal compression, and a left pleural effusion were noted (Fig. 3A). During the night prior to admission, she had complained of anterior neck and chest pain. While blood was being drawn for appropriate studies, she sustained a respiratory arrest. The child was successfully resuscitated and was transferred to the intensive care unit.

Physical examination revealed an afebrile child weighing 11.1 kg, who was breathing 40 times per minute. Although there was no cervical adenopathy, her neck was full and the suprasternal notch was not palpable. Intercostal retractions were present, and harsh inspiratory and expiratory rhonchi in addition to bilateral wheezing were heard. The liver and spleen were normal but a large mass was palpated in the left flank. A complete blood count, serum electrolytes, kidney and liver function studies, and serum uric acid levels were all normal. Bone marrow aspirate revealed no malignant cells. The intravenous pyelogram showed diffusely enlarged kidneys. Intravenous corticosteroids and allopurinol were begun, and within five days there was almost complete resolution of the mediastinal (Fig. 3B) and abdominal masses. Examination of cells obtained from a left thoracentesis

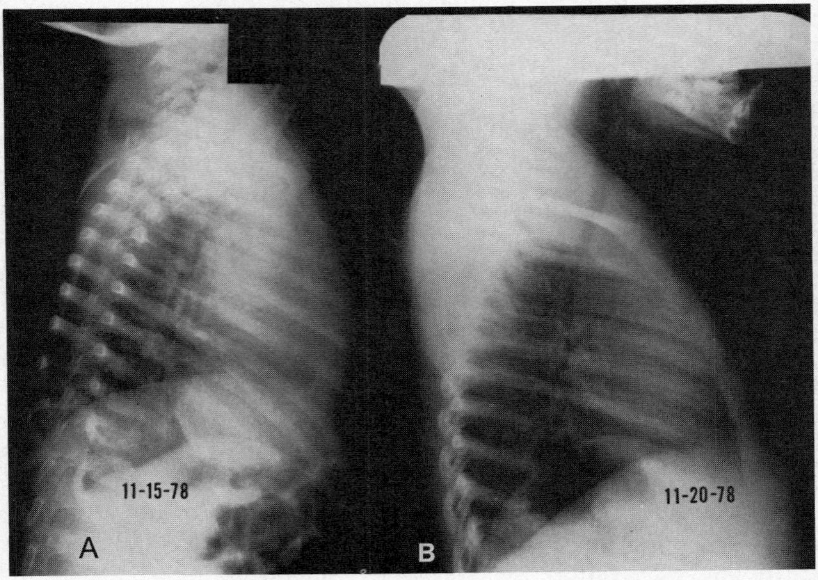

FIG. 3. Lateral films of the chest of a two-year-old girl. (A) Film obtained several days after the onset of respiratory difficulty. This shows an anterior mediastinal mass almost completely obliterating the airway. (B) Film obtained after five days of corticosteroid therapy. The airway is now patent, although the mediastinal mass is still present. These findings are characteristic of mediastinal non-Hodgkin's lymphoma.

showed E-rosette-forming convoluted lymphocytes (Fig. 4). The child was subsequently treated for non-Hodgkin's lymphoma involving the mediastinum and both kidneys; the therapy included multiple chemotherapeutic agents and radiation therapy.

PRIMARY LYMPHOMAS ORIGINATING IN LYMPH NODES, BONES, AND OTHER SITES

Enlargement of cervical, and occasionally supraclavicular, axillary, or inguinal lymph nodes is a frequent presenting physical finding in children with non-Hodgkin's lymphoma. The rapidity of growth and the magnitude of the lymphadenopathy should suggest NHL rather than Hodgkin's disease. Other symptoms include anorexia, cough, earache, fever, malaise, pain on swallowing, and weight loss. In early childhood, lymphoid tissue responds to infection with marked hyperplasia and, therefore, there may be a delay in diagnosis because of these nonspecific symptoms. While the pediatrician waits expectantly for resolution of the lymphadenopathy, either spontaneously or subsequent to treatment with antibiotics, the lymph nodes may enlarge or fail to regress.

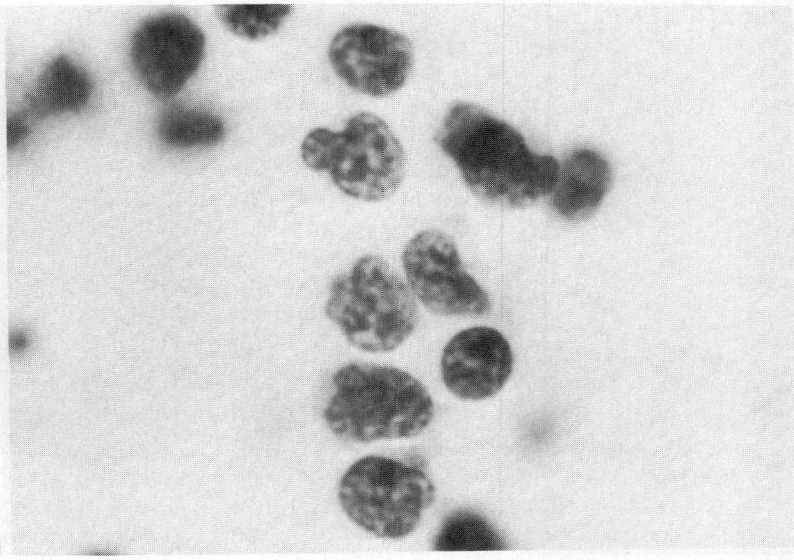

FIG. 4. Photomicrograph of cells obtained from thoracentesis in a patient with an anterior mediastinal mass causing respiratory distress. There are small immature lymphoid cells with convoluted nuclei and scant cytoplasm. (Wright's stain, reduced from ×1200)

Bone pain accompanied by localized swelling and tenderness is frequent in skeletal primaries. Tumors of the nasopharynx, paranasal sinuses and orbit are often accompanied by localized symptoms such as pain, nasal congestion, rhinorrhea, epistaxis, headache, and proptosis.

Lymph node primaries account for 15–45% of reported cases.[10,11,24,43] Again, there is a male predominance, and most cases occur during the early school years.[10] The majority present with advanced stage diseases,[10,27] often manifest by bone marrow involvement. Here the distinction between acute leukemia and non-Hodgkin's lymphoma is especially difficult. Regardless of the extent of bone marrow involvement, knowledge of the functional characteristics of the cells obtained from examining fresh tissue permits the selection of the most appropriate therapy and has the greatest likelihood of predicting the outcome. Skeletal primaries probably occur in less than 10% of patients,[11,28,43] although this group may also include patients with acute lymphocytic leukemia.[10]

Even if the bone marrow is not involved at the time of diagnosis, patients with lymph node involvement, especially those with generalized lymphadenopathy, are at significant risk for developing marrow involvement. In one large series, 57% of children with local or regional disease had leukemic conversion; the incidence of leukemic conversion increased to 84% when multiple lymph node sites were initially involved.[11] Between 20% and 40% of these children showed CNS involvement.[27,28] Skin primaries also have a high risk for marrow relapse and for subsequent CNS involvement.[44]

Published observations regarding the histological variants seen in lymph node and skeletal primaries suggest that the nodular lymphomas may be somewhat more frequent in head and neck primaries.[35,44] However, all histologic variants of non-Hodgkin's lymphomas, including Burkitt's lymphoma, lymphoblastic lymphoma, convoluted cell lymphomas, and follicular center cell lymphoma, have been described in lymph node primaries.[31,36,37,45,46] When surface marker studies have been performed, T, B, and null cells have been found.[38,39,46]

Prior to the widespread use of multiagent chemotherapy for non-Hodgkin's lymphoma, approximately 50% of children with localized head and neck primaries could be cured with combinations of surgery, irradiation, and single agent chemotherapy.[29,33,44] More recent reports suggest that the addition of multiagent chemotherapy has greatly improved the outlook for patients with either localized lymphoma or with widespread lymph node involvement.[10,27,42,47]

Improved survival in patients with skeletal primaries has not been as dramatic, except in the Boston series where six out of six patients with localized or regional bone involvement remain in continuous remission.[27] There is still a need for more effective therapy for advanced stage lymphomas originating from skeletal primaries.[10]

CONCLUSIONS

Children with non-Hodgkin's lymphoma often present with signs and symptoms characteristic of much more common diseases. Thus the diagnosis of NHL may be considered in children with enlarged lymph nodes, with respiratory distress, or with abdominal signs and symptoms. When the possibility of NHL is borne in mind, deliberate consideration can be given to the collection of fresh tissue or cells for examination for surface markers. These specimens can be obtained at surgery or from aspirates from the chest, abdomen, or bone marrow. Extent of disease as judged by the clinical presentation, bone marrow and spinal fluid findings, and functional characteristics of the malignant cells provide the essential criteria for selection of therapy and for predicting outcome.

References

1. Young JL Jr, Miller RW: Incidence of malignant tumors in U.S. children. *J Pediatr 86:254–258, 1975.*
2. Davies JNP: Some variations in childhood cancers throughout the world, in Marsden HB, Steward JK (eds): *Tumours in Children.* Springer-Verlag, New York, 1976, pp. 28–58.
3. O'Conor GT: Persistent immunologic stimulation as a factor in oncogenesis with special reference to Burkitt's tumor. *Am J Med 48:279–285, 1970.*
4. Marsden HB, Steward JK: Non-leukaemic reticuloendothelial tumours and leucosarcomas, in Marsden HB, Steward JK (eds): *Tumours in Children.* Springer-Verlag, New York, 1976, pp. 98–136.

5. Meadows AT, Jenkin RDT, Anderson J., *et al*: Irradiation and multiagent systemic chemotherapy utilizing moderate dose methotrexate for non-Hodgkin's lymphoma in children. *Med Pediatr Oncol 8(1), 1980.*
6. Kersey JH, Spectator BD, Good RA: Cancer in children with primary immunodeficiency diseases. *J Pediatr 84:263–264, 1974.*
7. Hoover R, Fraumeni JF Jr: Risk of cancer in renal-transplant recipients. *Lancet 2:55–57, 1973.*
8. Glatstein E, Goffinet DR: Staging of Hodgkin's disease and other lymphomas. *Clin Haematol 3:77–90, 1974.*
9. Murphy SB: Prognostic features and obstacles to cure of childhood non-Hodgkin's lymphoma. *Semin Oncol 4:265–271, 1977.*
10. Wollner N, Burchenal JH, Lieberman PH, *et al*. Non-Hodgkin's lymphoma in children; a comparative study of two modalities of therapy. *Cancer 37:123–134, 1976.*
11. Jaffe N, Buell D, Cassady JR, *et al*: Role of staging in childhood non-Hodgkin's lymphoma. *Cancer Treat Rep 61:1001–1007, 1977.*
12. Martin DJ, Ash JM: Diagnostic radiology in non-Hodgkin's lymphoma. *Semin Oncol 4:297–309, 1977.*
13. Horn NL, Ray GR, Kriss JP: Gallium-67 citrate scanning in Hodgkin's disease and non-Hodgkin's lymphoma. *Cancer 37:250–257, 1976.*
14. Ferrucci JT Jr: Body ultrasonography. *N Engl J Med 300:590–602, 1979.*
15. Rosenberg SA: Validity of the Ann Arbor staging classification for the non-Hodgkin's lymphomas. *Cancer Treat Rep 61:1023–1027, 1977.*
16. Carbone PP, Kaplan HS, Musshof, *et al*: Report of the committee on Hodgkin's disease staging classification. *Cancer Res 31:1860–1861, 1971.*
17. Wollner N: Non-Hodgkin's lymphoma in children. *Pediatr Clin NAm 23:371–378, 1976.*
18. Murphy SB: Current concepts in cancer; childhood non-Hodgkin's lymphoma. *N Engl J Med 299:1446–1448, 1978.*
19. Jenkin RDT, Sonley MJ, Stephens CA, *et al*: Primary gastrointestinal tract lymphoma in childhood. *Radiology 92:763–767, 1969.*
20. Zea JM, Exelby PR, Wollner N: Abdominal non-Hodgkin's lymphoma in childhood. *J Pediatr Surg 11:363–369, 1976.*
21. Murphy SB, Hustu HO: A randomized trial of combined modality therapy of childhood non-Hodgkin's lymphoma. *Cancer 45:630–637, 1980.*
22. Burkitt D: A sarcoma involving the jaws in African children. *Br J Surg 46:218–223, 1958.*
23. Pagano JS, Huang CH, Levine P: Absence of Epstein-Barr viral DNA in American Burkitt's lymphoma. *N Engl J Med 289:1395–1399, 1973.*
24. Hutter JJ, Favara BE, Nelson M, Holton CP: Non-Hodgkin's lymphoma in children; correlation of CNS disease with initial presentation. *Cancer 36:2132–2137, 1975.*
25. Nelson DF, Cassady JR, Traggis D, *et al*: The role of radiation therapy in localized resectable intestinal non-Hodgkin's lymphoma in children. *Cancer 39:89–97, 1977.*
26. Magrath IT, Lwanga S, Carswell W, Harrison N: Surgical reduction of tumour bulk in management of abdominal Burkitt's lymphoma. *Br Med J 2:308–312, 1974.*
27. Carabell SC, Cassady JR, Weinstein HJ, Jaffe N: The role of radiation therapy in the treatment of pediatric non-Hodgkin's lymphomas. *Cancer 42:2193–2205, 1978.*
28. Watanabe A, Sullivan MP, Sutow WW, Wilbur JR: Undifferentiated lymphoma, non-Burkitt's type; meningeal and bone marrow involvement in children. *Am J Dis Child, 125:57–61, 1973.*
29. Glatstein E, Kim H, Donaldson SS, *et al*: Non-Hodgkin's lymphoma. VI. Results of treatment in childhood. *Cancer 34:204–211, 1974.*
30. Rappaport, H: Tumors of the hematopoietic system, in *Atlas of Tumor Pathology,* Section 3, fascicle 8. Armed Forces Institute of Pathology, Washington, D.C., 1966.
31. Lukes RJ, Parker JW, Taylor CR, *et al*: Immunologic approach to non-Hodgkin's lymphomas and related leukemias; analysis of the results of multi-parameter studies of 425 cases. *Semin Hematol 15:322–351, 1978.*

32. Williams AH, Taylor CR, Higgins GR, *et al*: Childhood lymphoma-leukemia. I. Correlation of morphology and immunological studies. *Cancer 42:171–181, 1978.*
33. Pinkel D, Johnson W, Aur RJA: Non-Hodgkin's lymphoma in children. *Br J Cancer 31(Suppl. II):298–323, 1975.*
34. Jones B, Klingberg WG: Lymphosarcoma in children; a report of 43 cases and review of the recent literature. *J Pediatr 63:11–20, 1963.*
35. Wollner N, Lieberman P, Exelby P, *et al*: Non-Hodgkin's lymphoma in children; results of treatment with LSA_2-L_2 protocol. *Br J Cancer 31(Suppl. II): 337–342, 1975.*
36. Nathwani BN, Kim H, Rappaport H: Malignant lymphoma, lymphoblastic. *Cancer 38:964–983, 1976.*
37. Barcos MP, Lukes RJ: Malignant lymphoma of convoluted lymphocytes; a new entity of possible T-cell type, in Sinks LF, Godden JO (eds): *Conflicts in Childhood Cancer; An Evaluation of Current Management.* Alan R. Liss, New York, 1975, pp. 147—177.
38. Coccia, PF: Characterization of the blast cell in childhood non-Hodgkin's lymphoproliferative malignancies. *Semin Oncol 4:287–296, 1977.*
39. Jaffe ES, Braylan RC, Frank MM, *et al*: Heterogeneity of immunologic markers and surface morphology in childhood lymphoblastic lymphoma. *Blood 48:213–222, 1976.*
40. Kaplan, J. Mastrangelo R, Peterson WD Jr: Childhood lymphoblastic lymphoma, a cancer of thymus-derived lymphocytes. *Cancer Res 34:521–525, 1974.*
41. Weinstein HJ, Vance ZB, Jaffe N, *et al*: Improved prognosis for patients with mediastinal lymphoblastic lymphoma. *Blood 53:687–694, 1979.*
42. Murphy SB: Management of childhood non-Hodgkin's lymphoma. *Cancer Treat Rep 61:1161–1173, 1977.*
43. Murphy SB, Frizzera G, Evans AE: A study of childhood non-Hodgkin's lymphoma. *Cancer 36:2121–2131, 1975.*
44. Traggis D, Jaffe N, Vawter G, Baez-Biangreco A: Non-Hodgkin's lymphoma of the head and neck in childhood. *J Pediatr 87:933–936, 1975.*
45. Arseneau JC, Canellos, GP, Bansk PM, *et al*: American Burkitt's lymphoma; a clinicopathologic study of 30 cases. I. Clinical factors relating to prolonged survival. *Am J Med 58:314–321, 1975.*
46. Brunning RD, McKenna RW, Bloomfield CD, *et al*: Bone marrow involvement in Burkitt's lymphoma. *Cancer 40:1771–1779, 1977.*
47. Jenkin R, Anderson J, Chilcote R, *et al*: Grossly localized childhood non-Hodgkin's lymphoma (NHL): response to irradiation and elective four- or 10-drug combination chemotherapy (abstract). *Proc Am Soc Clin Oncol/Am Assoc Cancer Res 20:354, 1979.*

CHAPTER FIVE

Chemotherapy of Childhood Non-Hodgkin's Lymphoma

MARTIN MOTT, MB, MRCP

CHEMOTHERAPY IS THE MAJOR component of treatment for childhood non-Hodgkin's lymphomas (NHL), and it has greatly improved the prognosis for this group of disorders. To understand this dramatic change, it is necessary to review briefly the natural history of NHL and the historical evolution of treatment. Much of this information is contained in more detail in other chapters of this book.

NATURAL HISTORY

Non-Hodgkin's lymphomas differ markedly from Hodgkin's disease. Thus while Hodgkin's disease is a relatively indolent process and spreads by involvement of contiguous lymph nodes, neither of these statements is true of non-Hodgkin's lymphomas. Failure to appreciate these differences has caused an inordinate delay in the application of appropriate treatment.

The childhood non-Hodgkin's lymphomas also differ considerably from their adult counterpart, notably in their histological and anatomical distribution and in their clinical behaviour. Nodular histology of tumours is rare in childhood, more than 95% of tumours being of the diffuse variety, and the disease is systemic at the time of diagnosis in all but a small proportion of cases. Treatment strategies devised for adult tumours are largely irrelevant to children, and the significance of results from treating one group should only be extrapolated to the other with considerable caution.

NHL is clearly more than one disease entity. The lack of an appropriate classification at present only emphasizes the current state of confusion. There are, however, clear-cut patterns beginning to emerge.

Department of Child Health, Royal Hospital for Sick Children, St. Michael's Hill Bristol BS2 8BJ, England

Sternberg sarcoma is also called convoluted cell lymphoma, diffuse lymphoblastic lymphoma, and T cell lymphoma/leukaemia. It is a disease entity that typically affects adolescent males, who present with a mediastinal mass and generalized lymphadenopathy. The disease is exquisitely sensitive to corticosteroids and radiation, but almost always spreads to involve the bone marrow and meninges. The median survival was only eight months in all series before the recent advent of intensive combination chemotherapy.

Burkitt's lymphoma is a discrete geographical and clinical entity that is described in detail elsewhere in this book. It is a tumour of B cell lineage and is endemic in tropical Africa and New Guinea. It is clinically distinct from the so-called American Burkitt's tumours, which are usually abdominal B cell tumours, and may well be the same disease as those B cell tumours placed in the diffuse undifferentiated non-Burkitt's category.

Diffuse histiocytic lymphoma is a misnomer for a group of disorders of transformed lymphoid cells of various types. (They may consist of T, B, or null lymphocytes, or monocytes.)

EVOLUTION OF TREATMENT

The evolution of treatment for childhood non-Hodgkin's lymphomas mirrors that of most other childhood tumours and has resulted in the same delay in establishing an effective treatment regimen. In the era when surgical resection was the only available treatment, the proportion of patients with strictly localized disease who could be cured by surgery must have been very small. Radiation therapy has been available since the turn of the century. With the demonstration that it could cure some patients with Hodgkin's disease in the 1950s, efforts were made to copy this success in non-Hodgkin's lymphoma. The most that radiation can offer in this systemic disease of childhood, however, is to achieve an approximately 50% cure rate in the small minority of patients who present with localized disease; for example, 9 out of 22 patients in a recent report from Stanford.[1]

The modern era of successful treatment for childhood non-Hodgkin's lymphoma stems from the recognition that this is a disseminated disease in the great majority of patients, and therefore requires systemic treatment with chemotherapy. It is only in the recent past that chemotherapy has been applied, particularly to the treatment of adult non-Hodgkin's lymphoma. Until the late 1960s chemotherapy was used as single agent treatment, for example, cyclophosphamide or steroids, vinca alkaloids or procarbazine, and complete response rates of approximately 20% were achieved. A substantial improvement resulted from the combination of cyclophosphamide, vincristine, and prednisone (COP and CVP), these regimens being introduced by the National Cancer Institute and the Southwest Oncology Group (SWOG).[2,3] Adriamycin then became available and proved its worth as a single agent before being combined with COP to form CHOP.[4] The MOPP combination (nitrogen mustard, oncovin, prednisone, and procarbazine), which had proved highly successful in the treatment of Hodgkin's disease, was modified to C-MOPP and A-COPP. When bleomycin became available combinations such as CHOP-Bleo and BACOP were tested.[5,6] Other drugs recently found to be effective as single agents include the nitrosureas and epipodophyllotoxin.[7] Chemotherapy with single agents, or the standard adult combinations such as COP, have been relatively ineffective in childhood non-Hodgkin's lymphoma. The use of standard anti-leukaemia regimens has likewise been disappointing.[8,9]

The drug combinations currently in vogue are based on kinetic considerations, which are largely theoretically derived and of dubious clinical significance. An important concept in the formulation of such combinations is to provide an additive or synergistic effect against the tumour, while spreading the toxicity to normal tissues through various organ systems to an acceptable degree, thus improving the therapeutic ratio of the drugs. Most of the effective single agents against leukaemia and lymphoma are combined in doses and schedules that are given to maximum tolerance at approximately three-week intervals, allowing interim recovery from dose-limiting toxicities such as profound myelosuppression and immunosuppression.

BASIC CONCEPTS

Concepts that are basic to the current management of non-Hodgkin's lymphomas of childhood can be summarised as follows.

At least 80% of patients have generalized disease at diagnosis. Curative treatment therefore requires intensive combination chemotherapy. The primary role of surgery is to provide adequate tissue for a definitive histological diagnosis. It is possible that radiation may play an adjuvant role in the treatment of bulk disease where this is not managed more appropriately by surgery (for example, in gastrointestinal tumours after initial shrinkage by chemotherapy). Chemotherapy obviates the necessity for a vigorous search for microscopic disease outside of any planned radiation portal by surgical staging procedures. Though the Ann Arbor staging system appears to have some prognostic relevance in childhood non-Hodgkin's lymphoma,[1,16] it is of limited value because of the noncontiguous nature of dissemination and the high frequency of extranodal disease, especially involvement of bone marrow and meninges. Surgical staging is therefore irrelevant to the treatment of the great majority of patients and may cause a dangerous delay in the initiation of appropriate chemotherapy. The distinction between stage IV lymphoma with bone marrow involvement and leukaemia is largely one of semantics.

About half the 20% of patients with truly localized disease can be cured by radiation. It is not certain whether such children should receive chemotherapy in addition to radiation from the outset or if this should be introduced only if they later show evidence of relapse, since chemotherapy can probably salvage many patients who develop disseminated disease. In those patients with disseminated disease who receive radiotherapy as an adjuvant to chemotherapy, the dose and field of radiation should not be such as to limit systemic chemotherapy, but should aim primarily at helping to prevent local recurrence.

About one-third of patients develop evidence of central nervous system (CNS) disease. Meningeal infiltration is rarely the primary site of disease recurrence in patients with stage I and II disease, particularly those who have had complete resection of a gastrointestinal primary. It is at present recommended that all patients with more widespread disease should receive some form of prophylactic treatment to the CNS. There is some evidence that such prophylaxis is less effective in NHL than in leukaemia in preventing overt CNS involvement.[10,11]

THE PRESENT STATE OF THE ART

I will now review current results of the chemotherapy protocols that are being tested by a number of major groups and institutions.

Memorial Sloan-Kettering Cancer Center

The first indication that intensive combination chemotherapy had substantially altered the previously poor prognosis for childhood non-Hodgkin's lymphoma came from Memorial Hospital in New York.[10,12] In 1971 they modified their L2 leukaemia protocol and applied it to lymphoma patients. Treatment commenced with an initial high dose of cyclophosphamide and simultaneous radiation to bulk tumour. All patients then continued on an intensive induction, consolidation, and maintenance chemotherapy programme, which included intrathecal chemotherapy for CNS prophylaxis. Radiation was individualized, so that patients received doses ranging from 200 to 6200 rads, though many received no radiation at all.

By 1976 Wollner was able to report that 42 out of 58 patients (72%) were alive, 41 (70%) with no evidence of disease: 27 of the 42 survivors were off treatment, with a median survival of 45+ months.[10] Sixteen patients had died; 12 died of recurrence and dissemination and 4 died of viral infections. Seven out of 43 (16%) had developed evidence of CNS disease after diagnosis, despite use of prophylactic intrathecal methotrexate. However, only 1 out of the first 43 patients treated developed spread to the bone marrow while on treatment, though 19 patients (44% of the total) had bone marrow involvement at diagnosis and might, therefore, have been classified in other centres as patients with leukaemia. Only one out of nine children who presented with a mediastinal mass had developed evidence of recurrence.[11] The importance of adequate surgery in patients presenting with abdominal disease was emphasized in a separate report from the same group: 6 out of 7 survivors from a total of 31 patients had had complete resection of their tumour.[13]

A recent update of these figures recorded a disease-free actuarial survival of 95% at a median follow-up of 26 months among 61 patients considered to have been adequately treated.[14] It was acknowledged by these workers that such atment of childhood NHL is hazardous and requires very frequent and the use of all available supportive care.

ldren's Cancer Study Group

The Children's Cancer Study Group is currently examining in a randomized trial the relative therapeutic efficacy and toxicity of a modified LSA-L2 protocol against a less intensive protocol that includes cyclophosphamide, vincristine, methotrexate IV, and prednisone (COMP), together with radiation to bulk disease.[15] Results from 227 patients show that LSA-12 is superior for lymphoblastic histologies (particularly mediastinal presentations), while COMP is superior for diffuse undifferentiated histologies. This is clear evidence that chemotherapy strategy should be selective for different histologic subsets of childhood NHL.

Sidney Farber Cancer Institute

The Boston experience with childhood non-Hodgkin's lymphoma has recently been reported.[16] In this study 64 patients aged under 18 years were treated from January, 1971, to December, 1976, all patients with more than 5% of blasts in the bone marrow being excluded. Chemotherapy was variable during the first part of this time, but a standard regimen (APO) was used from 1973 to 1976. This regimen consisted of induction with prednisone, 40 mg/m^2 per day, vincristine, 1.5 mg/m^2 per week intravenously for four weeks, and adriamycin, 75 mg/m^2 on weeks one and four (except for patients with gastrointestinal primaries). Maintenance chemotherapy consisted of five-day courses of prednisone, 120 mg/m^2 per day, mercaptopurine, 225 mg/m^2 per day, with vincristine, 1.5 mg/m^2, and adriamycin, 30 mg/m^2 i.v. on day one to a cumulative adriamycin dose of 450 mg/m^2. Thereafter, methotrexate was substituted at a dose of 7.5 mg/m^2 daily for five days. The details of the concurrent radiation therapy protocol used are outside the scope of this review.

Actuarial five year survival for this series was 61% (disease-free survival 54%), ranging from approximately 90% in stage I to approximately 35% in stage IV. Survival for patients treated with APO (adriamycin, prednisone, and oncovin) was 78% compared with 50% before its introduction. All recurrences were within 19 months of diagnosis. Of nine patients with abdominal primaries treated since 1971 with a combination of surgery, radiation, and chemotherapy, seven are currently surviving.

A subsequent report from the same group on 12 children with initial mediastinal involvement treated by this chemotherapy regimen together with craniocervical radiation for CNS prophylaxis records an actuarial survival of 86% with a median follow-up of 41 months.[17]

St. Jude Children's Research Hospital

In the period from 1962 to 1975, 64 patients with childhood non-Hodgkin's lymphoma were treated, and 19 of these patients survived from 40 months to 10

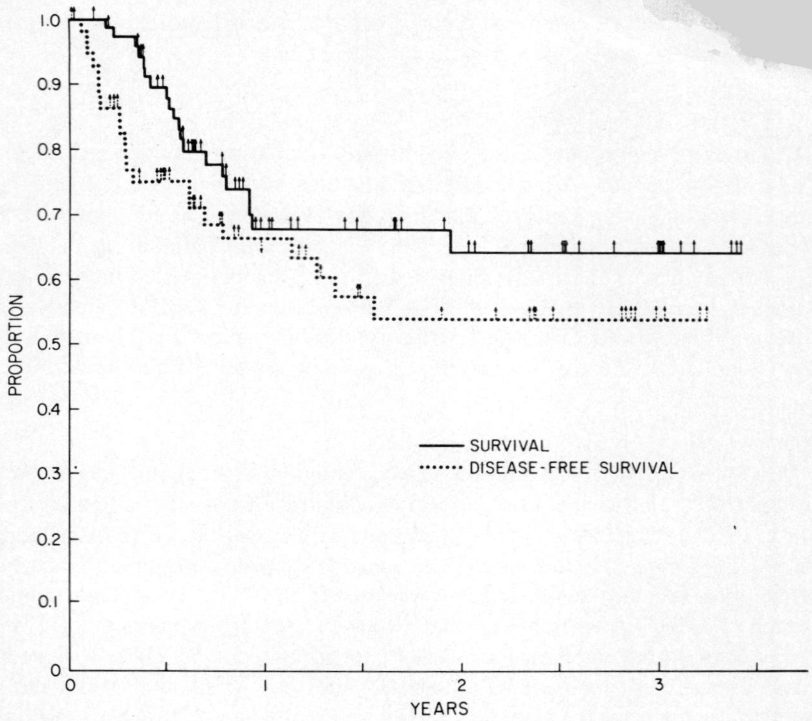

FIG. 1. Shown here (solid line) is the actuarial estimate of the proportion of all 69 patients entered in the study who are surviving, from diagnosis. Also shown (dotted line) is the actuarial estimate of the disease-free proportion of the 60 children achieving complete remission. Vertical bars indicate individual patients. (Reproduced with permission of Dr. S. Murphy and *Cancer*.)

years (30%). Seventeen of these 19 survivors (89%) were stage I or II at diagnosis.[18] A favourable subgroup of 25 patients presenting with localized disease between 1968 and 1975 were treated with a "total therapy" leukaemia programme together with involved field radiation. Twelve of these patients (48%) survived from 17 to 99+ months.

From March, 1975, to November, 1978, 69 patients entered a study designed to investigate the effectiveness of adjuvant radiation therapy to bulk tumour in patients with disseminated disease, and to assess the effectiveness of CNS prophylaxis with cranial radiation and intrathecal methotrexate.[19] Induction chemotherapy consisted of prednisone, 40 mg/m^2 per day for one month, vincristine, 1.5 mg/m^2 per week intravenously for six weeks, and cyclophosphamide, 1.2 gm/m^2 every three weeks for three doses. Patients with stage III and IV disease (St. Jude's staging), had in addition adriamycin, 45 mg/m^2, every three weeks for three doses. Patients with stage I and II disease had involved field radiation to a dose of 3000 to 3500 rad, whereas patients with stages III and IV

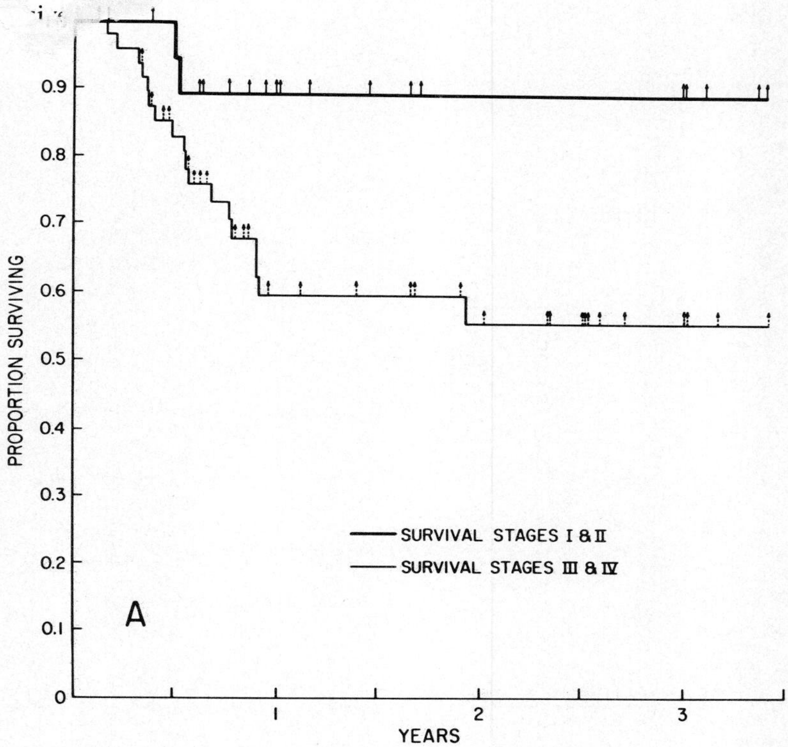

FIG. 2(a). The actuarial estimate of the overall survival for the 21 children with stages I and II disease is shown on the upper curve and compared to the estimate of overall survival of the 48 children with stage III and IV disease, shown in the lower curve.

disease were randomized to receive the same dose of radiation or no radiation to areas of bulk disease. All patients except those with stage I disease or stage II completely resected gastrointestinal primaries were randomized to receive 2400 rad cranial radiation plus intrathecal methotrexate, 12 mg/m^2 weekly for five doses, or no CNS prophylaxis. Maintenance chemotherapy was the same for all patients and consisted of mercaptopurine, 75 mg/m^2 per day, and methotrexate, 30 mg/m^2 per week, for 18 months.

Results of this study to date show a 90% two year disease-free survival for stage I and II disease (historically there was a 30% to 50% survival with radiation alone) and a 35% disease-free survival for stage III and IV disease[19] (Figs. 1 and 2). The addition of radiation in the latter group has so far shown no significant improvement (Fig. 3). There was, however, no evidence that the inclusion of radiation to bulk disease sites compromised the chemotherapy programme, which was relatively gentle compared to other regimens.

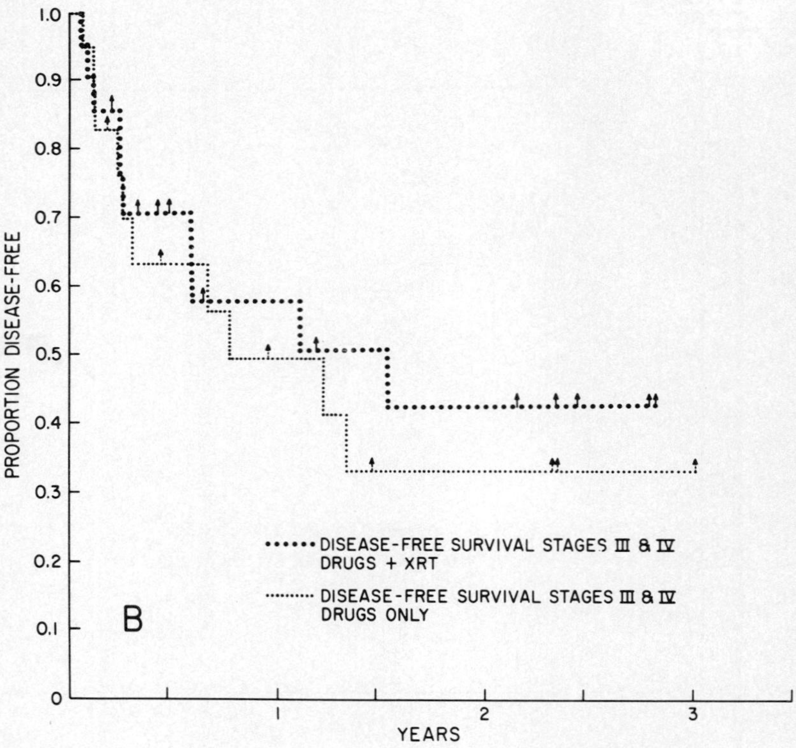

FIG. 2(b). The estimate of the disease-free survival for the 21 responding Stage I and II patients (upper curve) is shown in comparison to the actuarial estimate of the disease-free proportion of the 39 stage III and IV patients achieving a complete response (lower curve). Both the survival and the disease-free survival of the stage I and II patients are significantly better than that of stage III and IV patients ($p < 0.05$). (Reproduced with permission of Dr. S. Murphy and *Cancer*.)

Children's Hospital at Stanford

From May, 1975, to April, 1976, 12 patients entered a pilot study designed to test the efficacy of intensive combination chemotherapy as the primary treatment for childhood non-Hodgkin's lymphoma, with or without the addition of adjuvant low dose radiation to areas of bulk disease.[20] Nine of the 12 patients are surviving 34+ to 45+ months from diagnosis and 8 are in continuous complete remission. One patient with a mediastinal primary had a bone marrow relapse when off treatment at 32 months, but this patient is currently in remission at 45+ months. There have been three deaths; one in a patient who presented with involvement of multiple bones, one with a mediastinal primary and bone marrow involvement at diagnosis, and one who had previously treated disease and who entered the study after bone marrow relapse.

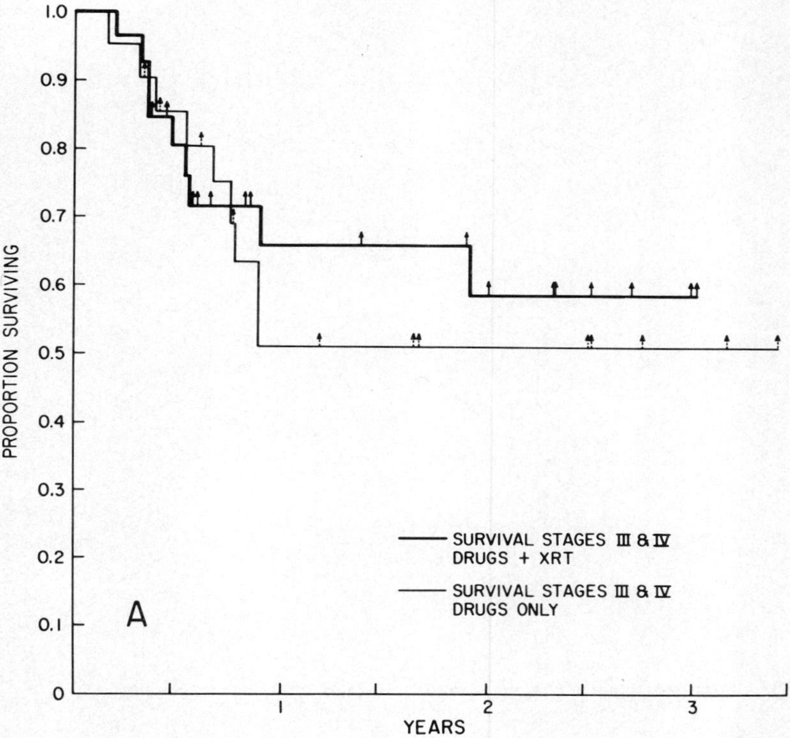

FIG. 3(a). The overall survival.

Of the six patients who presented with a mediastinal mass, five survive at 41+ to 45+ months with four in continuous complete remission.[21] Two of these four had no radiation, and two received 300 and 700 rad, respectively, to a localized area as emergency treatment for relief of respiratory and superior vena cava obstruction. The two patients who had bone marrow relapse at 27 and 32 months had received 450 rad to the mediastinum and 1500 rad to the mediastinum and right hemithorax, respectively.

United Kingdom Children's Cancer Study Group

Based on this pilot experience and that of other centres, the Stanford protocol was modified and has been used as the basis for a trial organized by the United Kingdom Children's Cancer Study Group (UKCCSG). The primary purpose of this trial is to confirm that intensive combination chemotherapy is the current treatment of choice in childhood non-Hodgkin's lymphoma, and to answer the question whether adjuvant low dose (1500 rad) radiation therapy to areas of bulk

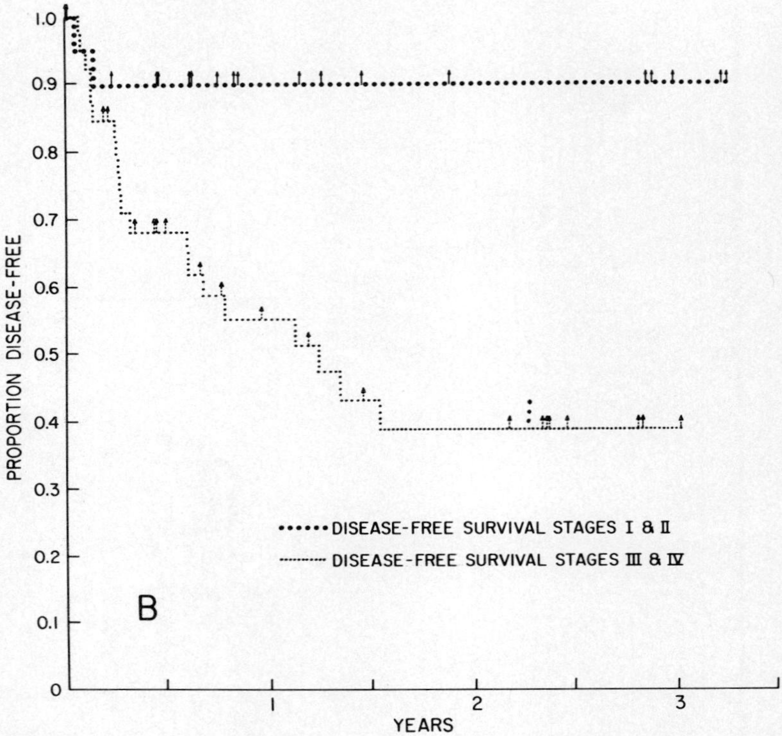

FIG. 3(b). The disease-free survival are shown above for the 46 children with stage III and IV disease who were randomised to receive either four drug combination drug induction only (no XRT) or the same four drugs plus involved field radiation therapy (XRT). There was no clinically or statistically significant ($p = 0.6$) benefit conferred by the addition of irradiation to bulky tumour in these advanced stage patients. (Reproduced with permission Dr. S. Murphy and *Cancer*.)

disease contributes anything further to such treatment. The treatment schedule is outlined in Tables 1 and 2 and in Fig. 4. The initial success of this programme, particularly for T cell lymphomas, has led to its further modification for use in patients with T cell leukaemia.

CONCLUSIONS

Much of the present confusion surrounding the management of this group of disorders stems from the failure to recognize the different diseases that masquerade under this name. It is quite clearly not the same disease as acute lymphoblastic leukaemia (ALL), so it is no surprise that standard antileukaemia treatment is

TABLE 1
United Kingdom Children's Cancer Study Group Protocol Design for Therapy of non-Hodgkin's Lymphoma (Stages II, III, and IV): Induction Regimen

Intensive combination chemotherapy, with or without radiation to areas of bulk disease		
Induction		
1. CHOP		
Cyclophosphamide	1 g/m^2	Day 1
Adriamycin	50 mg/m^2	Day 1
Vincristine	1.5 mg/m^2	Day 1
Prednisolone	100 mg/m^2	Days 1-5
	Given every three weeks for two cycles	
2. Cyt/TG		
Cytosine arabinoside	100 mg/m^2 intravenously or subcutaneously 12 hourly for 8 doses	
Thioguanine	75 mg/m^2 p.o. daily for 4 doses Given every three weeks for two cycles	
3. Intrathecal methotrexate	10 mg/m^2 (maximum 12 mg) on day 1 of each course	

relatively ineffective. On the other hand, T cell lymphoma is almost certainly the same disease as T cell leukaemia, for which standard ALL treatment is also inadequate. Since intensive combination chemotherapy, such as that outlined above, appears to be successful in the treatment of T cell lymphoma, it is logical to suggest that T cell leukaemia should be treated in a similar way.

The natural history of this group of diseases has changed in those given intensive combination chemotherapy as their primary treatment. Once the incidence of recurrence in bulk tumour, bone marrow, and central nervous system is known for patients with the various disorders given such treatment, the next step will be to develop more selective combination chemotherapy programmes for each group, with or without adjuvant surgery and radiation, according to need. This process of simplification and individualization will be our task for the 1980s. The present "blunderbus" approach to treatment is a necessary preliminary to a more selective era, for the first priority must be to increase the proportion of patients who are cured of their disease.

TABLE 2
United Kingdom Children's Cancer Study Group
Protocol Design for Therapy of Non-Hodgkin's Lymphoma
(Stages II, III, or IV): Consolidation and Maintenance Regimen

Consolidation

1. Methotrexate, 500 mg/m^2 (one-third i.v. push two-thirds i.v. drip over six hours)
2. 24 h after the beginning of the infusion, folinic acid 12 mg/m^2 i.m. or i.v. followed by three doses 6 mg/m^2 (i.v. or oral) over the next 24 h
3. Intrathecal methotrexate 10 mg/m^2 at the start of i.v. methotrexate infusion

Given every two weeks for three cycles

Randomization

With or without 1500 rad of radiotherapy to areas of bulk disease concurrently with consolidation chemotherapy

N.B. Special category for patients with Sternberg sarcoma

1. Methotrexate 15 mg/m^2 oral daily $\times$ 4 every 2 weeks $\times$ 3 instead of i.v. methotrexate
2. Intrathecal methotrexate on day 1 of each course
3. Cranial radiation, 1760 rad in eight fractions of 220 rad over two weeks

Maintenance

1. Cyclophosphamide/CCNU
   Cyclophosphamide 750 mg/m^2
   CCNU 75 mg/m^2 p.o.
2. VM 26 100 mg/m^2 intravenously

   Methotrexate 500 mg/m^2 intravenously with citrovorum factor rescue (as in consolidation)

   N.B. For patients with Sternberg sarcomas who have received cranial radiation, methotrexate will not be given i.v. but orally at a dose of 12.5 mg/m^2 daily for four days
3. CHOP
   Cyclophosphamide 750 mg/m^2
   (adriamycin 40 mg/m^2)
4. Cytosine arabinoside/thioguanine
   Cytosine arabinoside 150 mg/m^2 i.v. or s.c. } Daily $\times$ 5 days
   Thioguanine 75 mg/m^2 p.o. }

   Given at three week intervals. Twelve week maintenance cycle for two years.

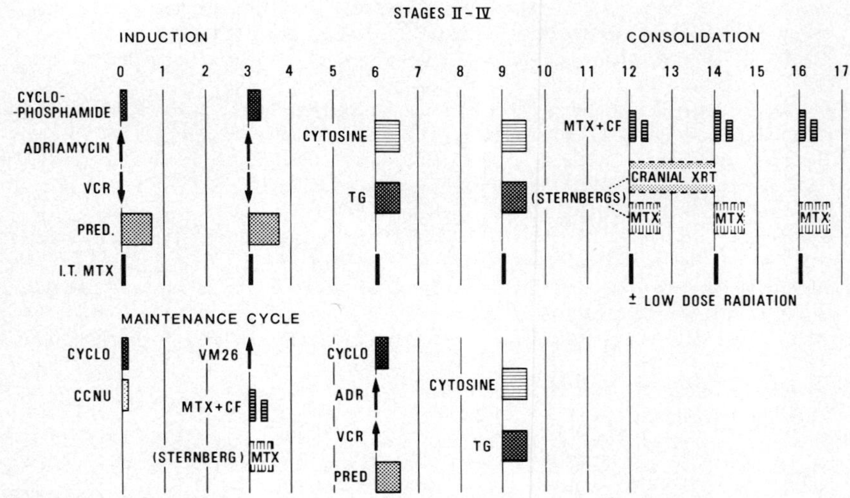

FIG. 4. Diagram summarising the UKCCSG protocol design for therapy of non-Hodgkin's lymphoma in children (stages II, III, and IV).

References

1. Glatstein E, Kim H, Donaldson SS, *et al*: Non-Hodgkin's lymphomas. VI. Results of treatment in childhood. *Cancer 34:204–211, 1974*.
2. Luce JK, Gamble JF, Wilson HE, *et al*: Combined cyclophosphamide, vincristine and prednisone therapy of malignant lymphoma. *Cancer 28:206–217, 1971*.
3. Bagley CM, De Vita VT, Berard CW, Canellos GP: Advanced lymphosarcoma; intensive cyclical combination chemotherapy with cyclophosphamide, vincristine and prednisone. *Ann Intern Med 76:227–234, 1972*.
4. Gottlieb JA, Gutterman JU, McCredie KB, *et al*: Chemotherapy of malignant lymphoma with adriamycin. *Cancer Res 33:3024–3028, 1973*.
5. Rodriguez V, Cabanillas F, Burgess MA, *et al*: Combination chemotherapy (''CHOP-Bleo'') in advanced (non-Hodgkin) malignant lymphoma. *Blood 49:325–330, 1977*.
6. Skarin AT, Rosenthal DS, Moloney WC, Frei E: Combination chemotherapy of advanced non-Hodgkin's lymphoma with bleomycin, adriamycin, cyclophosphamide, vincristine and prednisone (BACOP). *Blood 49:759–763, 1977*.
7. Bender RA, DeVita VT: Non-Hodgkin's lymphoma, in Staquet MJ (ed): *Randomized Trials in Cancer: A Critical Review by Sites*. Raven Press, New York, 1978.
8. Pinkel D, Johnson W, Aur RJA: Non-Hodgkin's lymphoma in Children. *Br J Cancer 31(Suppl. II):298–323, 1975*.
9. Cebrian-Bonesana A, Schwartzman E, Roca-Garcia C, *et al*: Non-Hodgkin's lymphoma in children; an analysis of 122 cases from Argentina. *Cancer 41:2372–2378, 1978*.
10. Wollner N: Non-Hodgkin's lymphoma in children. *Pediatr Clin N Am 23:371–378, 1976*.
11. Sullivan MP: Treatment of lymphoma. *Cancer 35:991–995, 1975*.

12. Wollner N, Burchenal JH, Lieberman PH, *et al*: Non-Hodgkin's lymphoma in children; a comparative study of two modalities of therapy. *Cancer 37:123–134, 1976.*
13. Zea JM, Exelby PR, Wollner N: Abdominal non-Hodgkin's lymphoma in childhood. *J Pediatr Surg 11:363–369, 1976.*
14. Wollner N, Jereb B: Multidisciplinary LSA_2-L_2 protocol treatment of non-Hodgkin's lymphoma in children; a review of 73 cases (abstract C-23). *Proc Am Soc Clin Oncol 20, 1979.*
15. Jenkin R, Anderson J, Chilcote R, *et al.*: Childhood NHL. Preliminary results of a randomized clinical trial (abstract C-262). *Proc Am Soc Clin Oncol 21, 1980.*
(abstract C-234). *Proc Am Soc Clin Oncol 19:365, 1978.*
16. Carabell SC, Cassady JR, Weinstein HJ, Jaffe N: The role of radiation therapy in the treatment of pediatric non-Hodgkin's lymphomas. *Cancer 42:2193–2205, 1978.*
17. Weinstein HJ, Vance ZB, Jaffe N, *et al*: Improved prognosis for patients with mediastinal lymphoblastic lymphoma. *Blood 53:687–694, 1979.*
18. Murphy SB: Management of childhood non-Hodgkin's lymphoma. *Cancer Treat Rep 61:1161–1173, 1977.*
19. Murphy SB, Hustu HO: A randomised trial of combined modality therapy of childhood non-Hodgkin's lymphoma. *Cancer 45:630–637, 1980.*
20. Wilson JA, Mott MG, Wilbur JR: Intensive combination chemotherapy of childhood non-Hodgkin's lymphoma (abstract C-202). *Proc Am Soc Clin Oncol 18:1977.*
21. Wilbur JR, Mott MG, Wilson JA: Childhood non-Hodgkin's lymphoma of the mediastinum; combination chemotherapy as primary treatment (abstract C-506). *Proc Am Soc Clin Oncol 20:414, 1979.*

CHAPTER SIX

Treatment of Non-Hodgkin's Lymphomas: Radiotherapy

ADRIAN R. TIMOTHY, MRCP, FRCR; JOHN E. FREEMAN, MRCP, FRCR

THE NON-HODGKIN'S LYMPHOMAS (NHL) are a heterogeneous group of diseases, characterized by differing clinical presentations and patterns of evolution. Unlike Hodgkin's disease, truly localized non-Hodgkin's lymphoma is uncommon and, when it does occur, frequently involves extranodal sites.[1] Comparison of non-Hodgkin's lymphoma in children and in adults reveals significant differences, which have important implications for the design of effective treatment programs.[2] For example, the high incidence of abdominal or mediastinal involvement in children is well documented,[3,4] whereas well-differentiated or nodular histological subtypes, associated with a more indolent natural history, are distinctly unusual in childhood.[5-7] Similarly, the frequent conversion to acute leukemia in childhood non-Hodgkin's lymphoma is in contrast to the relatively rare occurrence of this complication in adults.[8-11]

The majority of children with non-Hodgkin's lymphoma have either clinically apparent or occult dissemination of disease at the time of presentation, with subsequent involvement of the bone marrow or central nervous system being a common event. Thus it might be anticipated that local treatment alone would produce few long-term survivors. Until the early 1970s, local or regional irradiation constituted the major component of therapy for childhood non-Hodgkin's lymphoma, but in most patients the disease rapidly disseminated, with median survival times in the order of only six to nine months.[7,12,13] Overall survival figures in selected series before 1973 varied between 11% and 23%, with the best results being obtained in those children with clinically localized (stage I) disease, in whom over 50% remained alive for longer than three years.[3,13,14] Relapses after one year were uncommon and those surviving without evidence of disease at 24 months could be considered to be cured of their disease.

St. Thomas's Hospital, London SE1 7EH, England; University of Texas Health Sciences Center, San Antonio, TX 78205

The Rappaport histological nomenclature and Ann Arbor staging classification for Hodgkin's disease are often applied to non-Hodgkin's lymphomas. However, many consider this inappropriate in children. Comparison of studies relating to treatment of non-Hodgkin's lymphomas in children has been hampered by variations in staging schemes, histological classification, and treatment techniques.

It is clear that certain subgroups of patients with truly localized presentations, such as those in whom disease is confined to one lymph node group or those with localized gastrointestinal non-Hodgkin's lymphoma, are not commonly associated with progression to leukemia and have approximately 50% cure rates when treated by radiation therapy alone.[13] However, because this pattern of disease is seen in only a minority of patients and is still associated with a continued risk of relapse, use of adjunctive chemotherapy must be considered in all cases at the time of initial treatment. For the majority of patients, intensive systemic therapy is a prerequisite for long-term disease-free survival, since distant recurrence, with or without marrow or CNS relapse, is a frequent cause of failure following local irradiation alone.

Surgery, radiation therapy, and chemotherapy all have immediate and delayed effects on normal tissues as well as on malignant tissues. The complications of surgery are in general well understood and, for the most part, avoidable. There is also much information regarding morbidity due to therapeutic irradiation which affects particular organs and sites. There is also new information about the specific and nonspecific complications of the various chemotherapeutic agents. Improvement in survival following intensive therapy has increased the awareness of the long-term toxicity of certain combinations of therapeutic modalities. In 1959, D'Angio[15] drew attention to the potentiation of x-ray effects on normal as well as tumor tissues by dactinomycin. The improved tumor responses reported by this group naturally stimulated interest in the potential for such combined therapy. As a result, there is now an increasing volume of literature describing the modification of early and late radiation effects on critical normal tissues by a wide range of cytotoxic drugs, including alkylating agents, antimetabolites and antitumor antibiotics.[16] Such unfavorable combined effects include the apparently increased risk of developing second malignant neoplasms following intensive therapy for Hodgkin's disease[17] and the increased CNS toxicity of intrathecal methotrexate when given in combination with irradiation, as compared with either agent given alone.[18,19] Careful records of all immediate and delayed sequelae must be kept, therefore, as an essential part of any assessment of combined therapy.

LOCALIZED HEAD AND NECK PRESENTATIONS

Approximately one-half of patients presenting with localized disease in the head and neck may be cured by radiation therapy alone.[3,13] True local relapse is uncommon. Recurrence more commonly occurs at distant sites or as overt leukemia with or without CNS involvement. When disease is localized to one lymph node group or to Waldeyer's ring (stage I or IE), survival rates of between

55% and 70% are obtained with use of various combinations of surgery, radiation therapy, and single-agent chemotherapy.[12,13,20] Tumor doses of 4000 to 4500 rad given during an interval of 4½ to 5 weeks are adequate for control of local disease in the majority of adult cases. However, lower doses of radiation therapy are often given in children, depending on age or potential for enhanced toxicity with concurrent drug administration.[4,21]

Little information is available at present on the role of prophylactic radiation therapy to adjacent, clinically uninvolved, lymph node groups. However, the noncontiguous relapse pattern of this disease suggests that this would be unlikely to influence survival rates. Localized extranodal involvement, particularly with diffuse histological subgroups, is stated by Lemerle to have a better prognosis[14]; but this finding has not been confirmed in results from other series.[13,20] Excellent results are often obtained by treating localized disease with predominantly local therapy. Nonetheless, it is not possible on the basis of clinical presentation or histology to separate out with confidence those patients with truly localized presentations in whom systemic therapy may be omitted.

A current trial in the United Kingdom includes adequate pretreatment staging techniques and is designed to compare radiotherapy alone with radiotherapy and short-term combination chemotherapy. When completed, this study should define the usefulness of local radiation therapy for stage I disease. But, until further information is available, patients with apparently limited disease should probably receive intensive chemotherapy together with local radiation therapy.

GASTROINTESTINAL PRESENTATIONS

Approximately one-third of non-Hodgkin's lymphomas in children originate in the abdomen.[4] In one reported series, 22% of patients had primary involvement of the gastrointestinal tract, and an additional 18% had extensive disease of uncertain origin, involving the mesentery, retroperitoneum, and pelvis.[22] Primary gastrointestinal tumors most commonly arise in the terminal ileum, cecum, and ascending colon. It is of interest that, with such presentations, first relapse in the bone marrow or CNS is a rare event.[23,24] Even with an apparently complete resection, surgery alone is curative for only a very small proportion of patients, but the addition of whole abdominal irradiation resulted in long-term survival in over 80% of a small series of patients, reported by Jenkin *et al.*[25] Similar results were obtained by Nelson and colleagues in Boston, using a combination of surgery, whole abdominal irradiation, and systemic chemotherapy.[24] In their study, 8 out of 11 children (73%) remained disease-free for more than two years, compared with none out of four undergoing resection alone, and 6 out of 18 (33%) treated with resection and chemotherapy.

The high success rate obtained when whole abdominal radiation is given after surgery raises the question of whether it is necessary to give additional chemotherapy in cases with limited and resectable abdominal disease. As with chemotherapy, the smaller the residual tumor mass the more effective radiotherapy is likely to be. Thus the importance of adequate excision at the time of surgery is emphasized by data from the Memorial Sloan-Kettering Cancer Center.[26] Six out of seven survivors in the MSKCC series had apparent complete removal of their tumor at the time of surgery, whereas of those in whom more limited procedures were undertaken, only one patient survived, even when surgery was followed by irradiation and intensive chemotherapy.

Further confirmation of the importance of adequate initial surgery can be obtained from studies on abdominal Burkitt's lymphoma, where bulk tumor reduction has resulted in highly significant improvements in both duration of remission and overall survival.[27] The influence of gross tumor resection on the subsequent outlook for these children has led to the recommendation of "second look" operations following initial chemotherapy for unresectable disease. In these cases a good response to chemotherapy may permit subsequent excision of residual tumor.[8] If residual disease proves inoperable, surgical clips can define the disease, to permit more precise localized radiotherapy. Computerized transaxial tomography, with its ability to accurately demonstrate intraabdominal disease, provides an effective means of assessing the response to chemotherapy without immediate resort to further exploratory surgery. If there is no significant reduction in tumor size on CT scan, further surgical intervention is deferred and whole abdominal irradiation may be given.

From the point of view of potential radiation toxicity, it would seem desirable to reduce the volume irradiated in these patients to a minimum. However, the results of using more limited abdominal irradiation fields are much less satisfactory.[22,24] For the majority of children with widespread abdominal non-Hodgkin's lymphoma, the disease is unresectable at the time of presentation, and their outlook remains poor at the present time. For patients with more localized tumors, the optimum management is to perform as complete a resection as possible, followed by systemic chemotherapy with or without whole abdominal radiation. With appropriate protection of the kidneys and liver, radiation doses to the whole abdomen to a midpoint dose of 2500 rad given in 25 fractions are well tolerated. With intensive chemotherapy and whole abdominal irradiation, the local and systemic toxicity is so severe that radiation must be reduced to doses of 2000 rad given to multiple sites of gross involvement.

The Children's Cancer Study Group has recently published information on a prospective randomized study. This study was designed to compare the use of radiation to sites of bulk disease and use of either a four-drug program consisting of cyclophosphamide, vincristine, methotrexate, and prednisolone, or a modification of the LSA2-L2 regimen.[4] Both groups received CNS prophylaxis using intrathecal methotrexate.[28] The patient population was limited to those with disease involving either one or two adjacent lymph node regions, Waldeyer's ring, the gastrointestinal tract, or any localized extralymphatic site. Mediastinal presentations were excluded. At the last report on this study, all patients remained in initial continuous remission, with no difference between the two chemotherapy programs. The investigators, therefore, have stopped the more aggressive arm and continue with the four-drug regimen only. Further data from these studies will provide additional information about morbidity due to radiotherapy and chemotherapy. Results of these studies will also allow modifications to be made in radiation doses with reference to volume of tissue irradiated, the site of administration of radiotherapy, and the need to modify radiation doses when chemotherapy is given concurrently.

MEDIASTINAL PRESENTATIONS

Mediastinal involvement with non-Hodgkin's lymphoma has traditionally been associated with a grave prognosis. When treated by radiotherapy alone, the majority of patients rapidly developed bone marrow or CNS involvement.[7,13] The recent success of intermittent combination chemotherapy in producing long-term remissions in this group,[4,29] together with acknowledged toxicity of certain agents when administered together with radiation,[30] has led several workers to question the value of giving radiotherapy as a part of primary management. Weinstein and colleagues[29] employ cranial irradiation as part of CNS prophylaxis. However, they suggest that, for the majority of patients, local mediastinal irradiation should be reserved for those presenting with respiratory or venous obstruction, or those in whom the mediastinal component of the disease fails to regress, or progresses following initial chemotherapy. The excellent results with their APO regimen (adriamycin, prednisone, and Oncovin) support this approach. Others suggest that disease-free survival might be improved if radiotherapy is used during the induction phase of intensive chemotherapy regimens; but there is a real risk of significant drug dosage limitation due to combined toxicity.

ADVANCED DISEASE

The prognosis for children presenting with widespread involvement by non-Hodgkin's lymphoma has improved dramatically following the introduction of effective chemotherapy programs. Thus, reappraisal of the role of radiotherapy in advanced disease, from being a purely palliative procedure to being an integral part of potentially curative regimens, is now required. The LSA2-L2 protocol developed by Wollner *et al.*[4] employs radiotherapy given in varying doses to sites of bulk disease, that is, tumors greater than 5.0 cm in diameter, in combination with intensive systemic and intrathecal chemotherapy. This LSA2-L2 protocol has demonstrated a significant improvement in survival rate for children with stage III and stage IV non-Hodgkin's lymphomas. However, the hazards of increased toxicity due to added radiation, coupled with the risk of long-term somatic or genetic damage, emphasize the need for a firm conclusion on the value of radiation in obtaining and maintaining remission in such therapy programs.

Radiotherapy to large volumes of bone marrow at the time of chemotherapy, while possibly contributing to overall treatment effect by reducing tumor bulk, may also result in severe hematological depression, necessitating treatment delay and prejudicing the ultimate outcome. Murphy and Hustu, in a randomized study comparing involved field radiotherapy and chemotherapy with chemotherapy alone for children with stage III or stage IV non-Hodgkin's lymphomas, showed no significant improvement in survival for a small group (33 patients) when radiotherapy was added. At the same time, increasing toxicity was noted in the patients given combined treatment.[31] Another small study reported by Meadows *et al.*,[32] however, stated that toxicity was tolerable even when radiation therapy was given to bulk disease in conjunction with several chemotherapeutic agents, including high-dose methotrexate.

Randomized studies are currently underway to assess the contribution of radiation to induction and maintenance chemotherapy protocols. However, for the present, it is appropriate to consider giving radiation to all sites of bulk disease greater than 3.0 cm in diameter at the time of presentation. Where the volume to be irradiated is large and, therefore, competitive toxicity is likely, radiation therapy should be delayed if possible until initial induction chemotherapy has been completed and there is evidence of bone marrow recovery. Where the treated volume is small and, therefore, unlikely to prejudice hematological tolerance, cautious concurrent radiotherapy and chemotherapy may be given. The volumes treated and the radiation doses given can vary from patient to patient, and take account of direct and competitive toxicity to relevant critical organs. In many cases, an arbitrary dose limitation of 2000 rad is made to enable multiple sites of involvement to be treated with tolerable toxicity.

CNS PROPHYLAXIS AND TREATMENT

Although it is uncommon as a presenting feature or as a finding at the time of diagnosis, approximately one-third of children with non-Hodgkin's lymphoma will develop CNS involvement during the course of their disease.[23,33,34] The incidence of initial relapse in the CNS varies considerably with the original presentation. It has an extremely low incidence in stage I, yet 50% of patients with mediastinal disease may eventually develop meningeal involvement.[23,25] The overall incidence of CNS relapse is uncertain because, until recent years, many patients did not survive long enough to develop this complication. But with improved systemic therapy and prolonged survival, the CNS has become increasingly important as a potential relapse site.

CNS prophylaxis is therefore an integral and early part of most intensive treatment regimens. The dramatic influence of cranial irradiation and intrathecal methotrexate in reducing meningeal relapse in children with acute lymphoblastic leukemia is well established.[35] Several workers have shown the apparent effectiveness of intrathecal methotrexate in reducing primary CNS relapse in non-Hodgkin's lymphoma.[3,28,36] However, Wollner *et al.* still reported a 16% CNS relapse rate following prophylaxis with intrathecal methotrexate alone. The toxicity of both methotrexate and radiation to neural tissue is now well known, and this toxicity is increased if parenteral or intrathecal methotrexate is given concurrently with or following cranial irradiation.[18,19,37] The risk of these complications is acknowledged. However, the high risk of treatment failure due to the presence of occult disease in the CNS, and the apparent success of cranial irradiation with intrathecal chemotherapy or prophylaxis, recommends the use of CNS therapy in all children at high risk of CNS relapse.[29]

Certain clinical presentations are associated with a reduced risk of relapse in the CNS, such as limited abdominal lymphoma, solitary bone lesions, and isolated nodal involvement. It is possible that CNS prophylaxis may be omitted in these cases, or given with reduced doses as part of the primary treatment program. But further study with modern chemotherapy programs is required before a firm decision can be made on this point.

The grave prognosis for children with established meningeal involvement demands aggressive management.[2,3,31] Either craniospinal radiotherapy alone or cranial irradiation in combination with intrathecal chemotherapy will relieve symptoms and eradicate CNS disease in a proportion of patients. However, such involvement often occurs in the presence of active disease at other sites and cannot therefore be considered in isolation. Irradiation of the whole craniospinal axis to doses of 2400–3000 rad given in 12–15 fractions is considered adequate to eradicate microscopic foci of CNS lymphoma. But this amount of radiation therapy will be severely myelosuppressive, and will seriously limit subsequent systemic chemotherapy.

When CNS involvement produces symptoms and signs at the time of diagnosis, radiotherapy to the whole brain and upper cervical spine in combination with intrathecal methotrexate is required. Simultaneous involvement of a lower spinal segment may require selective local irradiation also, because intrathecal methotrexate is inadequate treatment for control of gross spinal meningeal disease. When meningeal relapse occurs during remission, at only a short interval after induction, the possibility of methotrexate resistance should be considered. In these cases, preference is given to the use of whole brain and spinal cord irradiation alone.

BONE INVOLVEMENT

Reimer *et al.*, in a review of lymphoma appearing in bone, concluded that the majority of patients with apparent primary lymphoma in bone had evidence of disseminated disease if they were thoroughly investigated. Therefore, he concluded that the patients require systemic treatment.[38] The results of the LSA2-L2 protocol at the Memorial Sloan-Kettering Cancer Center, in a small number of patients with skeletal primaries, gave an overall survival figure of 40% at 40 months.[4] It was also noted that chemotherapy alone does not induce complete tumor regression. Thus it was recommended that radiation be given to the primary site.

Treatment should initially be given to the whole length of the affected bone, with a boost to the site of obvious involvement to a tumor dose of 4500–5000 rad given during a period of five to six weeks.[39] Meticulous care should be exercised in planning radiotherapy to avoid unnecessary normal tissue damage. In the case of tumors of the extremities, it is necessary to prevent excessive fibrosis and to avoid edema by sparing irradiation of peripheral lymphatic pathways wherever possible.

BURKITT'S LYMPHOMA

The optimum dose schedules for all histological types of non-Hodgkin's lymphomas are not yet established.[40,41] However, in many patients local tumor control can be obtained with moderate doses of radiation (3000–4000 rad), given with conventional daily fractionation schedules, 150–200 rad per fraction, five days a week. Burkitt's lymphoma is a specific subtype of non-Hodgkin's lymphoma, characterized by its distinctive histological appearance,[42] clinical features, and rapid growth rate. Experience with radiotherapy in this disease is limited, but response to conventional fractionated radiotherapy is generally poor.[43]

The rapid cell turnover in Burkitt's lymphoma makes it an attractive model in which to test the radiobiological hypothesis that a reduction in time interval between individual radiation fractions, superfractionation, might lead to an improved therapeutic effect when tumor cells proliferate faster than those of the adjacent normal tissues. Norin and Onyango[43] have reported a significantly better complete response rate with three times a day fractionated radiotherapy, with no adverse early or late normal tissue effects. This approach demands further examination in non-Hodgkin's lymphoma treatment programs, in situations where rapidly growing tumors show resistance to chemotherapy, or in the treatment of tumor bulk at the time of initial induction therapy.[44]

With regard to CNS prophylaxis in Burkitt's lymphoma, one controlled study showed no benefit from cranial or craniospinal irradiation in preventing CNS relapse.[45] Likewise, the efficacy of intrathecal methotrexate alone is not yet confirmed.[46] In a more recent publication, Ziegler *et al.*[47] have demonstrated the value of intrathecal chemotherapy in achieving long-term remission in established CNS disease. This finding suggests that, for the present, both modalities should be used in prophylaxis, despite the possible risks of late sequelae.

SUMMARY AND CONCLUSIONS

Modern treatment policies for non-Hodgkin's lymphomas in children have emphasized use of intensive chemotherapy, with radiotherapy to localized disease in doses of 3500–4500 rad. Increased toxicity and sequelae may dictate lower doses at some sites of involvement.

In localized gastrointestinal presentations, the importance of complete surgical resection is stressed, followed by whole-abdominal irradiation. In cases with extensive abdominal disease, tumor regression after chemotherapy may permit "second look" surgery; excision of remaining tumor or local radiotherapy to sites of residual disease may then be performed. In mediastinal presentations, radiotherapy may be used for CNS prophylaxis, for cases with airway obstruction that cannot be managed with chemotherapy alone, or merely as an adjunct for chemotherapy.

For widespread disease, improved survival has followed the irradiation of bulk disease after prior intensive chemotherapy, using lower doses (2000 rad) with tolerable toxicity. CNS prophylaxis to groups at high risk, with cranial irradiation and intrathecal methotrexate, is considered more effective than intrathecal methotrexate alone. However, cranial irradiation is only of temporary palliative benefit in CNS relapse. Primary bone disease requires systemic chemotherapy and intensive irradiation of involved bone (4500–5000 rad), or lower doses to multiple sites of bone disease.

Finally, in localized Burkitt's lymphoma, superfractionation has achieved better local control than conventional fractionation schemes, with no increase in morbidity.

References

1. Peckham MJ: Radiation therapy of the non-Hodgkin's lymphoma. *Semin Hematol 11:41–58, 1974.*
2. Rosenberg SA, Diamond HD, Dargeon HW, *et al*: Lymphosarcoma in childhood. *N Engl J Med 259:505–512, 1958.*
3. Murphy SB, Frizzera G. Evans AE: A study of childhood non-Hodgkin's lymphoma. *Cancer 36:2121–2131, 1975.*
4. Wollner N, Burchenal JH, Lieberman PH, *et al*: Non-Hodgkin's lymphoma in children; a comparative study of two modalities of therapy. *Cancer 37:123–134, 1976.*
5. DeVita VT, Canellos GP: Treatment of the lymphomas. *Semin Hematol 9:193–209, 1972.*
6. Jones SE, Fuks Z, Bull M, *et al*: Non-Hodgkin's lymphomas. IV. Clinicopathologic correlation in 405 cases. *Cancer 31:806–823, 1973.*
7. D'Angio GJ, Mitus A, Evans AE: The superior mediastinal syndrome in children with cancer. *Am J Roentenol 93:537–544, 1965.*
8. Murphy, SB: Management of childhood Non-Hodgkin's lymphoma. *Cancer Treat Rep 61:1161–1173, 1977.*
9. Aur RJA, Hustu HO, Simone JV, *et al*: Therapy of localized and regional lymphosarcoma of childhood. *Cancer 27:1328–1331, 1971.*
10. Willoughby M: Chapter 7, this volume.
11. Grundy GW, Greagan ET, Fraumeni JF: Non-Hodgkin's lymphoma in childhood; epidemiological features. *J Natl Cancer Inst 51:767–776, 1973.*
12. Lemerle M, Gerard-Marchant R, Sancho H, Schweisguth O: Natural history of non-Hodgkin's malignant lymphomata in children. *Br J Cancer 31(suppl 2):324–331, 1975.*
13. Glatstein E, Kim H, Donaldson SS, *et al*: Non-Hodgkin's lymphomas. IV. Results of treatment in childhood. *Cancer 34:204–211, 1974.*
14. Lemerle K, Gerard-Marchant R, Sarrazin D, *et al*: Lymphosarcoma and reticulum cell sarcoma in children; a retrospective study of 172 cases. *Cancer 32:1499–1507, 1973.*
15. D'Angio GJ, Farber S, Maddock CL: Potentiation of x-ray effects by actinomycin D. *Radiology 73:175–177, 1959.*

16. Phillips TL, Fu KK: Quantification of combined radiation therapy and chemotherapy effects on critical normal tissues. *Cancer 37:1186–1200, 1976.*
17. Arsenau JC, Canellos GP, Johnson R, DeVita VT: Risk of new cancers in patients with Hodgkin's disease. *Cancer 40:1912–1916, 1977.*
18. Price RA, Jamieson PA: Central nervous system in childhood leukaemia. II. Subacute leukoencephalopathy. *Cancer 35:306–318, 1975.*
19. McIntosh S, Klatskin EH, O'Brien RC, *et al*: Chronic neurological disturbance in childhood leukemia. *Cancer 37:853–857, 1976.*
20. Traggis D, Jaffe N, Vawter G, Baez-Giangreco A: Non-Hodgkin's lymphoma of the head and neck in childhood. *J Pediatr 87:933–936, 1975.*
21. Lipton A, Lee BJ: Prognosis of stage I lymphosarcoma and reticulum cell sarcoma. *N Engl J Med 284:230–233, 1971.*
22. Jenkin RDT, Sonley MF, Stephens CA, *et al*: Primary gastro-intestinal lymphoma in childhood. *Radiology 92:763–767, 1969.*
23. Watanabe A, Sullivan MP, Sutow WW, Wilbur JR: Undifferentiated lymphoma, non-Burkitt's type; meningeal and bone marrow involvement in children. *Am J Dis Child 125:57–61, 1973.*
24. Nelson DF, Cassady JR, Traggis D, *et al*: The role of radiation therapy in localized resectable intestinal non-Hodgkin's lymphoma in children. *Cancer 39:89–97, 1977.*
25. Jenkin RDT: Radiation in the treatment of non-Hodgkin's lymphoma in children. *Semin Oncol 4:311–315, 1977.*
26. Zea JM, Exelby PR, Wollner N: Abdominal non-Hodgkin's lymphoma in childhood. *J Pediatr Surg 11:363–369, 1976.*
27. Magrath ST, Lwanga S, Carswell W, *et al*: Surgical reduction of tumor bulk in management of abdominal Burkitt's lymphoma. *Br Med J 2:308–312, 1974.*
28. Jenkin R, Anderson J, Chilcote R, *et al*: Grossly localized childhood non-Hodgkin's lymphoma; response to radiation and elective 4 or 10 drug combination chemotherapy (abstract). *Proc Am Soc Clin Oncol 19:354, 1978.*
29. Weinstein HJ, Zebulon BV, Jaffe N, *et al*: Improved prognosis for patients with mediastinal lymphoblastic lymphoma. *Blood 53:687–694, 1979.*
30. Newburger PE, Cassady JR, Jaffe N: Esophagitis due to adriamycin and radiation therapy for childhood malignancy. *Cancer 42:471–423, 1978.*
31. Murphy S, Hustu HO: A randomized trial of combined modality therapy in childhood non-Hodgkin's lymphoma (abstract). *Proc Am Soc Clin Oncol 19:364, 1978.*
32. Meadows AT, Hann H, Evans AE: Moderate dose methotrexate with other agents and radiotherapy for untreated childhood non-Hodgkin's lymphoma (abstract). *Proc Am Soc Clin Oncol 18:327, 1977.*
33. Pinkel D, Johnson W, Aur RJA: Non-Hodgkin's lymphoma in children. *Br J Cancer 31(suppl 2):298–323, 1975.*
34. Hutter J, Savara DE, Nelson M, Holton CP: Non-Hodgkin's lymphoma in children; correlation of CNS disease with initial presentation. *Cancer 36:2132–2137, 1975.*
35. Pinkel D, Simone J, Hustu HO: Nine years experience with "total therapy" of childhood acute lymphocytic leukemia. *Paediatrics 50:246–251, 1972.*
36. Freeman AI: Non-Hodgkin's lymphoma (abstract G-75). *Proc Am Soc Clin Oncol 17:255, 1976.*
37. Meadows AT, Evans AE: Effects of chemotherapy on the central nervous system. *Cancer 37:1029–1085, 1976.*
38. Reimer RR, Chabner BA, Young RC, *et al*: Lymphoma presenting in bone. *Ann Int Med 87:50–55, 1977.*
39. Carabell SC, Cassady JR, Weinstein HJ, Jaffe N: The role of radiation therapy in the treatment on pediatric non-Hodgkin's lymphomas. *Cancer 42:2193–2205, 1978.*
40. Fuks Z, Kaplan HS: Recurrence rates following radiation therapy of nodular and diffuse malignant lymphoma. *Radiology 108:675–684, 1973.*
41. Bush RC, Gospodaröwicz M, Sturgeon J, Alison R: Radiation therapy of localized non-Hodgkin's lymphoma. *Cancer Treat Rep 61:1129–1136, 1977.*

42. Berard C, O'Conor GT, Thomas LB, Torloni H: Histopathological definition of Burkitt's tumor. *Bull WHO 40:601–607, 1969.*
43. Norin T, Onyango J: Radiotherapy in Burkitt's lymphoma; conventional or superfractionated regime; early results. *Int J Radiat Oncol Biol Phys 2:399–406, 1977.*
44. Suit HD, Wette R: Theoretical considerations on the influence of dose fractionation on effectiveness of radiation therapy. Conference on Radiobiology and Radiotherapy. *National Cancer Institute Monograph 24, 225–247, 1967.*
45. Olweny CL, Atine E, Kaddu-Mukasa A, *et al*: Cerebrospinal irradiation of Burkitt's lymphoma. *Acta Radiol 16:225–231, 1977.*
46. Ziegler JL: Treatment results of 54 American patients with Burkitt's lymphoma are similar to the African experience. *N Engl J Med 297:75–80, 1977.*
47. Ziegler JL, Macgrath IT, Olweny CLM: Cure of Burkitt's lymphoma; ten year follow up of 157 Ugandan patients. *Lancet 2:936–938, 1979.*

CHAPTER SEVEN

Mass and Metabolic Effects of Non-Hodgkin's Lymphomas in Children

ELIZABETH KURCZYNSKI, MD; JOHN GRAHAM-POLE, MD, MRCP

UNTIL VERY RECENTLY the prognosis for children with non-Hodgkin's lymphoma has remained poor. A review of 64 children treated at St. Jude Children's Research Hospital between 1962 and 1973 recorded only 19 (30%) long-term survivors.[1] As discussed in detail elsewhere,[2-5] the use of refined diagnostic and staging procedures combined with application of intensive chemotherapy, plus radiation therapy to bulk disease and sanctuary sites, has dramatically improved the prognosis for these patients. Therefore, it is imperative that immediate complications both of the disease and of its treatment be recognized and corrected promptly and vigorously.

This chapter is concerned with two groups of well-recognized and extremely hazardous complications: (1) local pressure effects of large tumor masses at different sites, and (2) metabolic disturbances produced by the tumor and by its treatment.

MASS EFFECTS OF NON-HODGKIN'S LYMPHOMAS: PRESENTATION AND MANAGEMENT

Non-Hodgkin's lymphomas in children, particularly Burkitt's lymphoma, have such a rapid cell replication rate that sudden growth of large tumor masses may cause life-threatening symptoms requiring emergency treatment. Such symptoms include upper airway obstruction, superior vena cava syndrome, respiratory compromise from massive pleural effusion, bowel obstruction, bilateral renal involvement, expanding intracranial tumor and spinal cord compression. This section will discuss the emergency management of these complications of rapid tumor growth.

Department of Pediatric Hematology and Oncology, Rainbow Babies and Childrens Hospital, 2101 Adelbert Road, Cleveland, OH 44106, and School of Medicine, Case Western Reserve University, Cleveland, Ohio

Head and neck complications

Approximately 5–10% of children with non-Hodgkin's lymphoma present with primary involvement of the head and neck.[6,7] Sites include the orbit and maxilla, Waldeyer's ring, paranasal sinuses, salivary glands, larynx, thyroid, and scalp.[8]

Orbital non-Hodgkin's lymphoma is rare in children, but may produce a rapid threat to vision. Exophthalmos is the most common symptom, followed by swelling of the upper eyelid.[9] The most frequently involved organ is the lacrimal gland. Because of the danger to vision caused by compression of the optic nerve by a rapidly enlarging lymphoma, biopsy and complete evaluation should be performed as rapidly as possible. Immediate chemotherapy is the optimal treatment, since this produces rapid tumor response and avoids the risk of retinal damage from radiotherapy.

Paranasal sinus tumors usually cause asymptomatic facial swelling.[10] The patients may develop sudden signs of CNS involvement due to extension into the meninges via erosion of the posterior wall of the maxillary, ethmoid, or sphenoid sinus.[11] In this situation, immediate radiotherapy achieves rapid local tumor control without interfering with further diagnostic studies to determine the presence of spread elsewhere.

Tonsillar enlargement is a relatively common presentation of non-Hodgkin's lymphoma.[12] These patients develop dysphagia or signs of a pharyngeal mass. The absence of high fever, pain, or a high white count is sufficient to exclude the diagnosis of a peritonsillar abscess. These lesions are more often unilateral than bilateral. Excisional biopsy provides both tissue for diagnosis and immediate relief of upper airway obstruction. For the rare case where enough tumor cannot be removed surgically to allow a free airway, immediate radiotherapy and chemotherapy are indicated.

Crouplike symptoms of inspiratory stridor plus a barking cough are the initial symptoms of non-Hodgkin's lymphoma involving the larynx.[13] Biopsy via direct laryngoscopy allows removal of sufficient tumor to relieve acute respiratory distress. Chemotherapy must be started early to prevent the known rapid regrowth of tumor.

Chest complications

Mediastinal lymph nodes are commonly involved in childhood non-Hodgkin's lymphoma. Twenty-two percent of Wollner's series of 86 children from the Memorial Sloan-Kettering Cancer Center had a mediastinal primary.[16] The superior mediastinal syndrome (SMS) is diagnosed when compression of superior mediastinal structures compromises the child's airway, and constitutes a medical emergency. Symptoms are venous engorgement, cyanosis, edema of the head and neck, stridor, dyspnea, cough, fever and chest pain. In a series of 124 children reported from Boston, 6% presented with superior mediastinal syndrome.[15] A lymphomatous etiology of this syndrome must be differentiated from neuroblastoma. Neural crest tumors affect younger children and usually involve the posterior mediastinum.

The problem of obtaining a tissue diagnosis in mediastinal non-Hodgkin's lymphoma has been discussed in Chapter 3 of this book. Children with SMS have severe respiratory compromise and cannot tolerate extensive diagnostic or surgical procedures. However, a tissue diagnosis can usually be made without performing a major surgical procedure. Thus biopsy of supraclavicular or cervical nodes (which are involved in 75% of these cases[16]), bone marrow aspiration and biopsy, or aspiration of an associated pleural effusion will often supply the diagnosis without the need for general anesthesia. A diagnosis of non-Hodgkin's lymphoma can be presumed when a child with the typical clinical picture of SMS responds dramatically to intravenous corticosteroids, but the opportunity for precise tissue diagnosis is then lost.[2] The likely diagnostic and therapeutic benefit of thoracotomy must be carefully weighed against the anesthetic risk, by the pediatrician, surgeon, and anesthesiologist.

Whether or not tissue is obtained initially, the child should be started immediately on chemotherapy to relieve the airway obstruction.[17,18] Local radiotherapy (three or four daily doses at 200 rad per dose) is also recommended, in order to produce maximum tumor shrinkage rapidly. Airway swelling may increase 4–6 h after the first x-ray treatment, but can be minimized by concurrent corticosteroid therapy given in high doses intravenously. These patients must be watched carefully, preferably in an intensive care unit, since emergency tracheostomy may be needed to maintain an airway.

Malignant pleural effusions frequently accompany mediastinal non-Hodgkin's lymphoma. If the fluid accumulation is large enough to cause dyspnea when the patient lies on his back, thoracentesis will relieve symptoms rapidly with minimal trauma to the child. Once radiotherapy and chemotherapy are initiated, the effusion usually resolves and repeated thoracenteses are rarely necessary.

Acute myocardial infarction has been reported in children due to myocardial infiltration by lymphoma.[19] This rare complication is usually diagnosed only at autopsy, but should respond to standard chemotherapy if the diagnosis is suspected on clinical grounds.

Abdominal complications

Complications are common with abdominal presentations of childhood non-Hodgkin's lymphoma. Any abdominal organ may be involved, as shown in Table 1. In this series of 81 children with primary abdominal presentations, 24 had either stage III or stage IV disease at the time of diagnosis.[20] Their presenting signs included pain, vomiting and diarrhea, fever, and a palpable mass (Table 2).

Surgery is frequently indicated for immediate management of abdominal lymphoma because of acute bowel obstruction. Non-Hodgkin's lymphoma is the most frequent cause of intussusception in children over six years of age and is much

TABLE 1
Primary Sites of Abdominal Non-Hodgkin's Lymphoma in Children[a]

Location of primary	Number of patients
Small bowel	49
Appendix	10
Colon	8
Ovary	6
Kidney	3
Meckel's diverticulum	2
Stomach	2
Liver	1
Total	81

[a]Adapted from Zea *et al.*[20]

more common in boys. These children usually show the classic triad of cramping abdominal pain, bloody stools, and a palpable mass, but the diagnosis is often delayed because intussusception is an uncommon problem beyond infancy.[21,22] The surgeon must be alert to the possibility of lymphoma before emergency surgery is performed, because complete excision of these tumors improves the prognosis. In addition, lymph node and liver biopsies must be performed, as well as a thorough search of the abdomen for other sites of tumor involvement.

If the child's abdominal symptoms do not require immediate surgery, several new diagnostic techniques are helpful in defining the extent of disease. Computed tomographic (CT) scanning correctly diagnosed the presence or absence of lymphoma in 85% of an adult series.[23] Lymphangiography may guide the surgeon in

TABLE 2
Initial Signs and Symptoms of Children with Abdominal Non-Hodgkin's Lymphoma[a]

Initial sign or symptom	Number of patients
Pain	23
Vomiting and diarrhea	11
Fever	6
Palpable mass	6
Anorexia	5
Abdominal distention	4
Weight loss	3
Intussusception	1
Acute GI bleeding	1
Ascites	1

[a]Adapted from Zea *et al.*[20]

selecting which lymph nodes to biopsy.[24] However, we have found lymphangiography to be of limited value because of technical problems in performing the procedure, because of difficulties in interpreting the results, and because it is contraindicated in patients with respiratory impairment. CT scanning and ultrasound together give accurate and rapid preoperative information about the extent of abdominal disease. In the rare case where a child is too sick to undergo laparotomy, peritoneoscopy offers a quick way to obtain biopsy tissue at minimal risk.[25]

The following case summary illustrates problems that may arise in a child with extensive abdominal non-Hodgkin's lymphoma.

> *Illustrative Case 1.* This five-year-old boy was admitted to the hospital in November, 1977, with a one-week history of abdominal cramps and blood-streaked stools. Initial examination was negative, but four days later a 10×10-cm pelvic mass was palpable. Initial blood counts, bone marrow biopsy, and spinal tap were normal. Chest film showed a massive right-sided pleural effusion. Barium enema revealed a large pelvic mass with upward displacement of bowel (Fig. 1). Biopsy of the abdominal mass showed a poorly differentiated lymphocytic lymphoma, Burkitt's type.
>
> The patient was started on combination chemotherapy. Within four days the abdominal mass was no longer palpable, and the patient was completely asymptomatic. Five days after discharge he was readmitted with a temperature of 38°C, and a recurrence of the abdominal mass. His hematocrit was 22%, white cell count 200/mm^3 with no polymorphonuclear leukocytes. Blood culture grew *Escherichia coli*. The patient was treated successfully with antibiotics and neutrophil transfusions, but he developed hypertension and azotemia due to renal artery compression by tumor. Radiotherapy to his right flank cleared these signs in five days. Over the next three months, the child was asymptomatic, but abdominal ultrasound showed a persistent 2×5-cm flank mass; thus chemotherapy was continued.
>
> Five months after diagnosis, the patient developed a right anterior chest wall mass and a recurrent right pleural effusion. He also had complete bone marrow replacement by tumor, liver metastases, invasion of the fourth lumbar vertebra, and malignant cells in his spinal fluid. Uric acid was 11.0 mg/dl, hematocrit 31%, white cell count 3000/mm^3 with 4% malignant cells and 82% polymorphs. He was begun on a course of total body irradiation which caused rapid but temporary symptomatic improvement. The child died 10 days later with respiratory failure and progressive disease.

Such complicated problems require the combined skills of the pediatric surgeon, radiotherapist, and pediatric oncologist. Although complete surgical removal of the tumor offers the best prognosis, chemotherapy must not be delayed by unnecessarily vigorous surgery, since residual tumor may regrow exceedingly rapidly, as occurred in our patient. Short courses of radiotherapy usually relieve bowel or renal obstruction, without causing enough marrow suppression to delay chemotherapy. Curative doses of radiotherapy are not required, because intensive

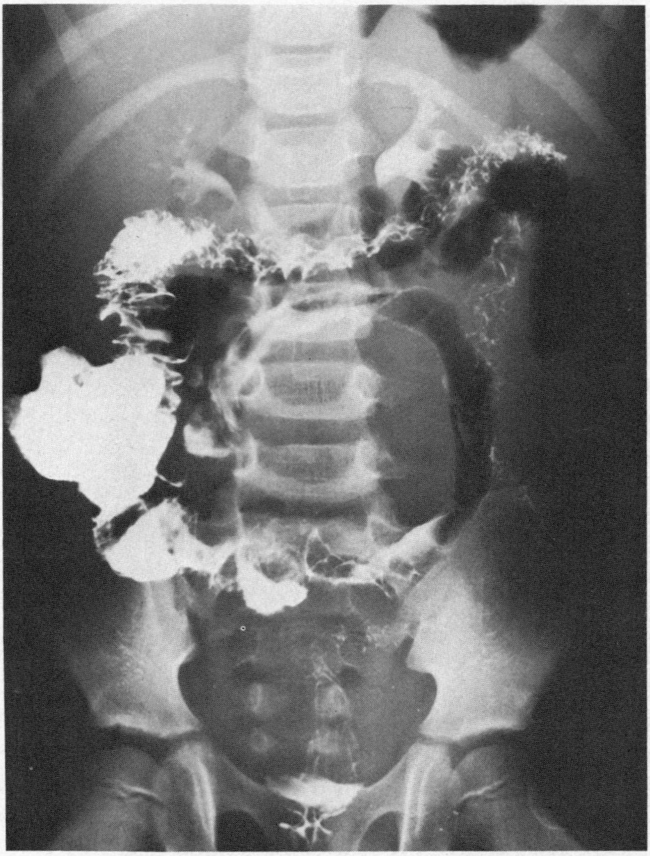

FIG. 1. Illustrative case 1. Barium enema at time of diagnosis showing displacement of bowel by a large midabdominal mass.

chemotherapy can control residual abdominal tumor with less accompanying toxicity.[26] The role of radiotherapy for treatment of extensive abdominal disease is discussed elsewhere in this book.[4] When radiation and chemotherapy are used together, however, there is an increased risk of cystitis when cyclophosphamide is used and an increased risk of enteritis from the combined use of adriamycin and abdominal radiotherapy.

Ovarian primary sites are not uncommon in non-Hodgkin's lymphoma in children. As in the case of intussusception, the surgeon should consider the possibility of finding lymphoma, so that adequate resection of the primary, as well as careful node biopsies and exploration for tumor spread, can be performed at the time of the initial operation.

CNS complications

The central nervous system is involved by non-Hodgkin's lymphoma in as many as 30% of children and usually presages a fatal outcome.[27] CNS involvement is most common in children who have mediastinal disease at diagnosis, particularly if there is also bone marrow involvement.[28,29] Diffuse meningeal involvement, analogous to that which occurs in acute leukemia, is less common now that most treatment regiments for non-Hodgkin's lymphoma include CNS prophylaxis.[29,30] Symptoms of intracranial involvement include headache, vomiting, cranial nerve palsies, and sudden weight gain. The diagnosis is confirmed by finding malignant cells in the spinal fluid.

Rapid clearing of the CSF and relief of symtoms may be achieved with intrathecal chemotherapy with methotrexate alone or by the use of "triple therapy," which consists of intrathecal methotrexate, cytosine arabinoside, and hydrocortisone. In addition, cranial irradiation may be given at a dose of 1800–2400 rad to the whole brain. It is not yet clear whether radiotherapy to the whole neuraxis can eradicate lymphoma once it is established in the CNS. Skarin reported that five out of six adult patients with lymphoma, who had CNS involvement refractory to other therapy, responded to high-dose intravenous methotrexate followed by folinic acid "rescue."[31] Although experience is limited, there is suggestive evidence that effective CNS prophylaxis in childhood non-Hodgkin's lymphoma may be achieved by giving a course of high-dose intravenous methotrexate together with intrathecal methotrexate.[32]

Paraplegia is an acute emergency that can occur in non-Hodgkin's lymphoma due to extradural spinal metastases. The radicular arteries become obstructed by tumor in retroperitoneal or retropleural spaces, thus producing ischemia of the spinal cord,[33] or tumor may extend directly to the cord through intervertebral foramina.[34] Most patients present with back pain, followed by weakness of varying severity. Numbness, paresthesias, leg cramps, and bladder or bowel problems are common. The spectrum of symptoms varies with the level of the compression, as outlined in Table 3.[35] Roentgenograms of the spine frequently show a paraspinous mass or involvement of adjacent vertebrae. If plain films fail to show the involved site, myelography is indicated to define the level of intraspinal block. Since this procedure may not show the full extent of the lesion if a complete block is present, a cisternal puncture may also be necessary. Spinal fluid is easily obtained at the time of myelography and usually shows malignant cells plus an elevated protein level.

Spinal cord compression tends to occur late in the course of lymphoma but it is occasionally a presenting symptom. The following case is typical.

> *Illustrative Case 2.* This 16-year-old white male presented in 1976 with enlarged cervical lymph nodes and a 6-lb weight loss. Biopsy of a cervical node revealed a poorly differentiated lymphocytic lymphoma. Complete evaluation showed no evidence of tumor spread. While he was receiving mantle radiotherapy, his counts dropped significantly, due to complete bone

TABLE 3
Clinical Localization of Spinal Compression[a]

Clinical localization	Spinal cord	Conus medullaris	Cauda equina
Vertebral level	Above T10	T10 to L2	Below L2
Motor impairment	Symmetric, profound weakness	Symmetric, mild to moderate weakness	Asymmetric, rarely severe
Tendon reflexes	Increased	Increased knee jerk, decreased ankle jerk	Asymmetric, decreased
Plantar response	Abnormal	Normal or abnormal	Normal
Sensory abnormalities	Symmetric, level common	Symmetric, saddle distribution	Asymmetric, dermatomal
Sphincter	Late	Early	Late, maybe absent

[a]Adapted from Baten and Vannucci.[35]

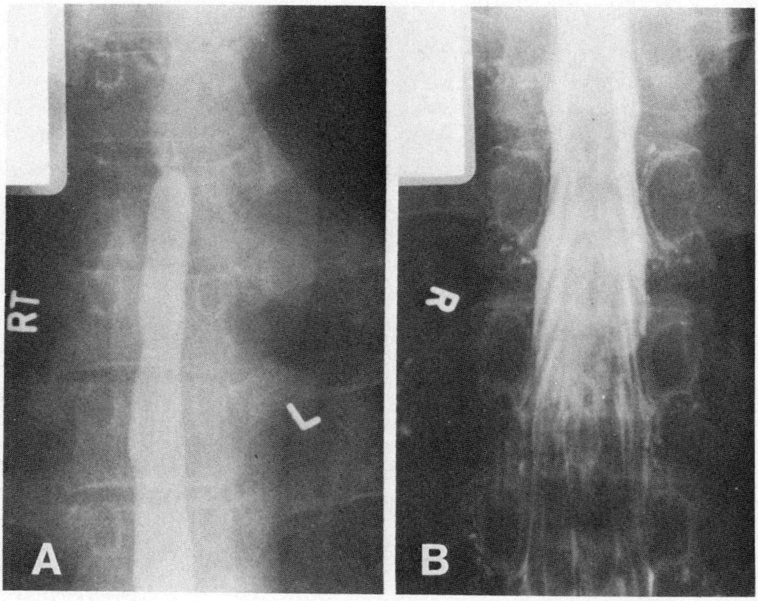

FIG. 2. Illustrative case 2. (A) Myelogram showing complete obstruction to CSF flow at C6. (B) Myelogram demonstrating partial obstruction by a mass at the cauda equina level, plus thickening of the cauda nerve roots by tumor involvement.

marrow replacement by tumor cells. He was treated with vincristine and prednisone every three weeks for one year, when chemotherapy was discontinued.

In July, 1978, he developed a pain in his right shoulder, which radiated down to his elbow and finger tips. Physical examination showed decreased sensation in the distribution of the right median nerve. Myelogram showed a large defect on the right side at the level of C5 and C6 vertebrae, with almost complete obstruction of CSF flow (Fig. 2). A laminectomy and tumor biopsy were performed and the histologic findings confirmed recurrence of the lymphoma. The boy was given 2000 rad to the involved cervical region plus chemotherapy, which caused complete resolution of symptoms.

Three months later he developed pain and weakness in his right leg plus constipation and hesitancy on urination. Physical examination revealed tenderness over the region of L4 and L5 vertebrae, back pain on straight leg raising, an absent right knee jerk, and decreased rectal sphincter tone. Myelogram showed a mass at the cauda equina level (Fig. 2). He was treated with radiotherapy but did not show improvement.

Although this patient received suboptimal treatment by current standards, he illustrates the many problems that arise from spinal or paraspinous involvement in non-Hodgkin's lymphoma. The cervical compression was treated promptly and effectively even though treatment could have been started without the delay of a biopsy. The cauda equina compression had progressed further, resulting in bowel and bladder involvement, which had become unresponsive to therapy.

The most effective treatment of sudden spinal cord compression by lymphoma is immediate radiotherapy. Usually, a total dose of 3000 rad given in increments of 150–200 rad to the involved area will produce rapid improvement.[36] Emergency decompression surgery can almost always be avoided, since these tumors are very sensitive to radiation. We give dexamethasone, at a dose of 8.0 to 16.0 mg per day in four to six divided doses, to reduce the cord swelling that may occur at the beginning of therapy. The steroid can usually be discontinued after seven to ten days if the child's symptoms are improving.

Prompt diagnosis of spinal cord involvement is the most important prognostic factor for its complete resolution. Clinicians must be alert to investigating thoroughly complaints of limping, extremity weakness, or back pain in children. In Friedman's series of 18 adults and children with cord compression due to non-Hodgkin's lymphoma, 65% showed complete recovery with radiotherapy.[37] If symptoms have progressed to loss of sphincter control, chances of recovery are poor.[37]

METABOLIC EFFECTS OF NON-HODGKIN'S LYMPHOMA: ETIOLOGY, PATHOLOGY, AND MANAGEMENT

Illustrative Case 3. A 16-year-old white girl was admitted to the hospital because of a mass in the left maxillary region, cervical lymphadenopathy and middorsal pain. There was rarefaction on roentgenographic examination of the vertebral bodies of T6 to T10. Initial laboratory studies included complete blood count, bone marrow aspirate and biopsy, and urinalysis, all of which were normal. The only biochemical abnormality was a serum uric acid of 8.3 mg/dl. Lymph node biopsy was diagnostic of Burkitt's lymphoma. The girl was treated with cyclophosphamide, vincristine, prednisone, intrathecal methotrexate, and radiation therapy to the facial and spinal lesions.

After initial improvement, she was readmitted six weeks later with generalized weakness, vomiting, and low back and limb pain. She was dehydrated and had abdominal masses. Her bone marrow showed leukemic transformation. There were widespread osteolytic lesions on skeletal survey, and intravenous pyelography revealed diffuse bilateral renal enlargement. Laboratory studies showed: serum sodium 136 mEq/liter, potassium 4.9 mEq/liter, chlorides 90 mEq/liter, bicarbonate 20 mEq/liter, calcium 11.8 mg/dl, phosphorus 5.7 mg/dl, blood urea nitrogen 30 mg/dl, creatinine 1.1 mg/dl, uric acid 16.2 mg/dl, lactic acid dehydrogenase (LDH) 2940 mU/ml. She was given intravenous fluids that included 200 mEq sodium bicarbonate given over a period of 24 h (to maintain the urinary pH above 7.0) and allopurinol, 800 mg/day, plus further combination chemotherapy.

Seventy-two hours later she was somnolent and her urinary output measured only 380 ml per 24 h. Laboratory values were: calcium 16.1 mg/dl, phosphorus 6.7 mg/dl, blood urea nitrogen 45 mg/dl, creatinine 2.6 mg/dl, uric acid 11.8 mg/dl, potassium 5.4 mg/dl, bicarbonate 17 mEq/liter. She received mithramycin at a dose of 25 mcg/kg given during four hours, which was repeated 48 h later. She also received intravenous isotonic saline and radiation therapy to the kidney to a total dose of 500 rad. Four days later her urine output had risen to 2000 ml per 24 h, serum calcium was 11.8 mg/dl, phosphorus 4.6 mg/dl, blood urea nitrogen 38 mg/dl, creatinine 1.7 mg/dl, and uric acid 6.8 mg/dl. The patient maintained a good partial remission on chemotherapy for four months; then she developed recurrent involvement of the bone marrow, bone, and abdomen. Once more the relapse of lymphoma was associated with elevated calcium (peak 13.8 mg/dl), phosphorus (peak 6.2 mg/dl), uric acid (11.0 mg/dl), and LDH (2160 mU/ml).

This girl had a combination of metabolic problems resulting from the rapid dissemination of her Burkitt's lymphoma to the bony skeleton, bone marrow, and kidneys. The primary event was probably an obstructive uropathy produced by the combined tumor infiltration and hyperuricemia.[39] Her renal insufficiency was probably aggravated by her rapidly developing hypercalcemia associated with an elevated serum phosphate level. These metabolic problems were rapidly reversed by combining direct treatment of the tumor using radiation therapy and chemotherapy, together with vigorous measures to control her hyperuricemia and hypercalcemia. Similar metabolic problems developed during later widespread recurrence of her disease.

HYPERURICEMIA

Etiology, pathology, and clinical picture

Virchow in 1851 first observed hyperuricemia and uricosuria complicating leukemia.[40] This has since been recognized as a common complication of malignant diseases, particularly cancers of the blood forming organs.[41-44] The incidence of this complication is much greater since the widespread use of effective chemotherapy and radiation therapy.

Uric acid is the final product in the degradation of nucleic acid purines, which are oxidized to hypoxanthine, xanthine, and uric acid, by the enzyme xanthine oxidase. Hyperuricemia arises in neoplasia both from accelerated proliferation and turnover of malignant cells and from their rapid destruction by cytotoxic therapy. It may, therefore, develop spontaneously and even before the diagnosis of lymphoma or leukemia is made[45,46]; but more often it follows upon rapid tumor cell destruction produced by treatment.[42,47,48]

The most frequent and dangerous consequence of hyperuricemia in malignant disease is acute uric acid nephropathy.[44,49,50] Other complications seen in more chronic disorders associated with hyperuricemia include renal calculus formation[41,49] and gouty arthropathy.[51] These complications are uncommon in cancer patients. Although hyperuricemia is seen following treatment of many forms of cancer, acute nephropathy seems to complicate only hematologic malignancies.[44,52] Raised serum uric acid levels lead to increased glomerular filtration and secretion of urates.[53] If the limited renal capacity for excreting urates is exceeded, urates precipitate in the lumen of the distal tubules and collecting ducts, causing back pressure upon the glomeruli. There may also be a direct toxic effect of uric acid on tubular epithelial cells.[54]

In blood at pH of 7.4 uric acid is largely in the form of the more soluble sodium urate, whereas uric acid itself predominates in acid urine. At a urine pH of 5.0, the solubility of uric acid is approximately 15 mg/100 ml, but this solubility increases to 200 mg/100 ml at pH 7.0.[53,54] Factors that influence the severity of nephropathy are the magnitude and duration of hyperuricemia, the magnitude and rate of tumor cell lysis, the degree of hydration and the urinary pH,[53] the presence or absence of coexisting renal disease (particularly lymphomatous or leukemic infiltration),[52,55] and the simultaneous presence of metabolic disturbances such as hyperphosphatemia and hyperkalemia.[49,50] Patients with Burkitt's lymphoma have a very rapid tumor cell turnover rate and often respond dramatically to chemotherapy. These patients are at particular risk for the severe metabolic consequences of massive tumor cell lysis.[5,50,56]

Typically, symptomatic hyperuricemia occurs in a patient with newly diagnosed lymphoma or leukemia, who has widespread disease in the form of bulky tumor masses and/or heavy bone marrow infiltration, which produces a high circulating blast cell count. Anorexia, nausea, and vomiting with consequent dehydration are common symptoms. Oliguria may progress to anuria with increasing renal insufficiency. Rarely, renal calculi cause colic and hematuria.[41,49] Severe weakness, somnolence, coma, and convulsions have been reported in leukemic children with hyperuricemia,[57] but these symptoms may also be attributable to coexistent metabolic disturbances such as hypocalcemia,[58,59] or primary CNS pathology. Most children with non-Hodgkin's lymphoma are at risk for developing symptomatic hyperuricemia because of their rapid cell proliferation and because they frequently have widespread dissemination at the time of diagnosis.

Treatment

In Table 4 treatment of uric acid nephropathy is divided into prevention and treatment of overt disease. Initial assessment must include: (1) blood pressure, (2) serum for uric acid, BUN, electrolytes, creatinine clearance, calcium and phosphorus, and (3) urinalysis for pH, blood, protein, and casts. Serum chemical determinations and urinalysis should be repeated frequently during the initial phases of treatment, particularly if biochemical abnormalities develop. An intravenous pyelogram is recommended to detect evidence of lymphomatous infiltration, obstructive uropathy, or other renal pathology.

TABLE 4
Management of Uric Acid Nephropathy

A. Preventive: for hyperuricemia
   1. Frequent biochemical profile: blood urea nitrogen, serum sodium, potassium, chlorides, calcium, phosphorus, bicarbonate, creatinine, uric acid; urine pH, electrolytes, and uric acid.
   2. Correct dehydration and maintain fluid balance, 3000 ml/m^2 5% dextrose in normal saline.
   3. Urinary alkalinization, pH greater than 7.0, sodium bicarbonate, 100-200 mEq/m^2/day. Acetazolamide, 250-500 mg/m^2/day.
   4. Allopurinol, 300 to 600 mg/m^2/day.
   5. Avoid uricosuric agents, salicylates, diuretics.

B. Therapeutic: for established nephropathy
   1. Attempt osmotic diuresis: mannitol, 25 gm/m^2, may repeat once.
   2. Consider cystoscopy to relieve obstructive sludge.
   3. Peritoneal dialysis or hemodialysis.

These children often have malaise and have diminished fluid intake. Intravenous fluids are recommended to correct dehydration and to maintain fluid balance, using 5% dextrose and half-normal saline together with replacement of other electrolytes as indicated. Careful input/output measurements are essential. As stated earlier, urate solubility is improved by alkalinizing the urine. Sodium bicarbonate in a dose of 100–200 mEq/m^2/day should maintain the urine pH between 7.0 and 8.0. Acetazolamide (Diamox), at a dose of 250–500 mg/m^2/day, can be initiated at the same time. This drug has both diuretic and uricosuric properties and promotes urinary alkalinization,[60] but it may aggravate systemic acidosis by inhibiting hydrogen ion excretion.

Allopurinol (Zyloprim) is a substrate for and a competitive inhibitor of the enzyme xanthine oxidase; xanthine oxidase catalyzes the conversion of hypoxanthine and xanthine to uric acid.[53,61] Allopurinol is now used routinely in the prophylaxis and treatment of hyperuricemia complicating lymphoma and leukemia.[47,55] Toxicity is minimal though severe hypersensitivity is reported, and xanthine may also accumulate to clinically significant amounts (see below). A dose of 300–600 mg/m^2 of allopurinol reliably reduces serum uric acid levels, but for maximum effect it should be started at least 24 h before beginning anticancer therapy. Allopurinol also potentiates the action of 6-mercaptopurine, which is degraded by xanthine oxidase. To avoid excessive myelotoxicity, the dose of 6-mercaptopurine should be reduced to 25% if it is given concurrently with allopurinol.[61] Cytotoxic agents, antibiotics, and other drugs with known nephrotoxic side effects should be used cautiously in hyperuricemic patients. Salicylates and thiazide diuretics tend to increase uric acid levels and furosemide lowers urinary pH. Thus all these drugs should be avoided.

If renal insufficiency develops in spite of these measures, osmotic diuresis should be attempted with mannitol, given at a dose of 25 g/m^2. Mannitol is given rapidly and repeated in an hour if there is no effect.[62] Cystoscopy and ureteral lavage may be appropriately used in the presence of renal colic, hematuria, and uric acid crystalluria. If these measures fail, and there are life threatening metabolic disturbances such as hyperkalemia, acidosis, and hyperphosphatemia, renal dialysis should be instituted. Though peritoneal dialysis may be effective for this complication,[63] hemodialysis is the treatment of choice, since it is 10 to 20 times more efficient than peritoneal dialysis in removing uric acid.[49] Use of hemodialysis also simplifies the patient's fluid, nutritional, and drug management.[50]

XANTHINURIA

Treating hyperuricemia by xanthine oxidase inhibition with allopurinol causes the oxypurines, xanthine and hypoxanthine, to accumulate. Xanthine excretion may rise as high as 150 mg/liter/day, which is equal to its solubility at a urinary pH of 5.0.[64] There have been a few reports of both adults and children with lymphoma who developed renal xanthine stones,[64,65] although no systematic study has been performed of the incidence of significant xanthinuria in these patients. Orotic acid and orotidine excretion is also increased in patients being treated with allopurinol.[66]

Treatment of xanthine nephropathy is by avoidance of excessive allopurinol, maintenance of a high volume of alkaline urine and, if necessary, use of hemodialysis. These oxypurines can be measured in urine and plasma by thin-layer chromatography or by spectrophotometry in patients at particular risk, such as children with disseminated Burkitt's lymphoma.[65]

HYPERCALCEMIA

Etiology, pathology, and clinical picture

Hypercalcemia is defined as serum calcium repeatedly above 11.5 mg/dl. It is a common complication of lung, renal, and breast cancer, and of multiple myeloma.[67,68] It is infrequent in other hematologic cancers, the incidence in non-Hodgkin's lymphomas being less than 5% in several series.[68,71] However, there are several reports of children with lymphoma developing severe hypercalcemia,[72,73] and it is a potentially lethal hazard that requires prompt recognition and treatment, as illustrated in the case report above. The protean clinical features of hypercalcemia are listed in Table 5.

Several mechanisms for production of hypercalcemia may be operative. The most common causative mechanism is the osteolytic effect of widespread skeletal metastases,[74,75] but hypercalcemia also occurs in the absence of overt bone or bone

TABLE 5
Clinical Features of Hypercalcemia

A. Gastrointestinal symptoms
   1. Anorexia
   2. Vomiting
   3. Abdominal pain
   4. Constipation

B. Neuropsychiatric symptoms and signs
   1. Muscle weakness
   2. Hyporeflexia
   3. Depression
   4. Obtundation
   5. Coma
   6. EEG: diffuse slow waves

C. Renal symptoms and signs
   1. Polyuria
   2. Polydipsia
   3. Calculi
   4. Renal insufficiency

D. Other findings
   1. Bone pain
   2. Pruritus
   3. Ocular and periarticular calcification

marrow involvement.[69,76] Suggested mediators include parathormone (PTH) or parathormonelike substances,[77,78] prostaglandin-E2,[79,80] specific osteoclast activating factor,[81] or an imbalance of normal humoral factors controlling skeletal and mineral homeostasis.[82] Ectopic parathormone production simulating primary hyperparathyroidism is a rare cause of hypercalcemia in lymphoma[77,83]; levels of immunoreactive parathormone are more often normal or low.[73,76,84] Prostaglandins seem to mediate hypercalcemia in certain solid tumors, both in animal models[79] and in human studies,[80] by increasing cyclic-AMP activity in bone and stimulating osteoclastic bone resorption. However, three hypercalcemic patients with non-Hodgkin's lymphoma had normal levels of prostaglandin metabolites as well as normal parathormone levels.[80] A peptide termed osteoclastic activating factor (OAF), which has potent bone resorbing activity, has been demonstrated in supernatants from three Burkitt's lymphoma cell lines.[81] To date this substance has only been found in cells of hematologic origin.[81,85,86] However, assessment of the importance of OAF as a mediator of hypercalcemia in lymphoma or leukemia must await its further characterization and reliable methods for *in vivo* measurement.

The ionized and albumin-bound fractions of calcium in the plasma are in constant equilibrium. Increase in the ionized proportion alters the excitability of cell membranes in nervous tissue as well as in skeletal muscle and smooth muscle.

TABLE 6
Guidelines for Management of Hypercalcemia

A. General treatment modalities
   1. Rehydration with normal saline
   2. Forced diuresis with furosemide or ethacrynic acid
   3. Renal dialysis
   4. Anticancer therapy

B. Specific medications
   1. Phosphate, oral or intravenous
   2. Corticosteroids
   3. Mithramycin
   4. Calcitonin

Widespread ectopic calcification may develop in the kidneys, in blood vessels, endocardium, intestinal mucosa, and lung, particularly when there is coexistent azotemia and hyperphosphatemia.[87] Effects on the kidney include both reduced glomerular filtration rate and renal tubular damage, as manifested by diabetes insipidus, salt wasting, and renal tubular acidosis. The level of serum calcium in hypercalcemic cancer patients is usually greater than 14 mg/dl, and serum calcium levels above 16 mg/dl constitute a medical emergency. Biochemical changes frequently associated with hypercalcemia are hypercalciuria, a normal or high serum phosphate, high alkaline phosphatase, high bicarbonate, hyperkalemia, and hypochloremia. There may be associated hyperuricemia and evidence of increased renal insufficiency.[68,74,88]

Treatment (Table 6)

Treatment is dictated by the nature of the underlying neoplasm (Table 6), which in these children is usually advanced with widespread skeletal involvement.[73,75] Treatment is also dependent on the severity of symptoms, the level of serum calcium, and the coexistence of other metabolic disturbances and of renal impairment.[50,58,79] Rehydration expands the intravascular compartment and increases the glomerular filtration rate. Intravenous isotonic saline, given at a rate of 3000 ml/m^2/day, both improves glomerular filtration and promotes calciuresis because of the closely related handling of calcium and sodium ions in the renal tubule.[89] Forced diuresis using furosemide (100 mg every one to two hours) or ethacrynic acid (20–40 mg every one to two hours) increases calcium excretion[68,90] by inhibiting sodium and calcium reabsorption at the level of the proximal tubule. Suki *et al.*[90] recorded a mean fall of serum calcium of 3.1 mg in eight patients; but they emphasized the need to maintain glomerular filtration by adequate hydration. Hemodialysis using a low calcium gradient may be effective in lowering the serum calcium level in refractory hypercalcemia.[91] Specific treatment measures for hypercalcemia include (1) oral or intravenous phosphate, (2) corticosteroids, (3) mithramycin, and (4) calcitonin.

1. *The use of oral or intravenous phosphate.*[88,92] Intravenous infusion of 50–100 mosmol of phosphate produced mean falls of serum calcium of 2.4–6.1 mg/dl in 24 h, accompanied by a fall in renal calcium excretion.[92] The probable action of phosphate administration is to lower the serum calcium level by increasing the skeletal calcium pool. Extraosseous calcification[87] and precipitous hypocalcemia[93] are serious hazards of phosphate administration. Such treatment requires careful monitoring, but it may be indicated in the presence of established renal dysfunction.[68] Alkalinization of the urine to combat coexistent hyperuricemia increases the risk of renal calcification with calcium phosphate.

2. *Corticosteroids.* These drugs are effective in the treatment of hypercalcemia complicating myeloma and breast cancer[67] and are a rational part of the therapeutic regimen for children with non-Hodgkin's lymphoma. Their hypocalcemic action is probably through inhibition of bone reabsorption, but they may also influence intestinal absorption and renal excretion of calcium.

3. *Mithramycin.* This antineoplastic antibiotic effectively lowers serum calcium in patients with malignant disease, with or without bony metastases.[72,76,94] It probably works by inhibiting osteoclastic bone resorption.[95] An intravenous infusion of 25 mcg/kg, which may be repeated up to a total dose of 150 mcg/kg/week, produces its hypocalcemic effect within 48 h.[96] Possible side effects of mithramycin are thrombocytopenia and hepatocellular necrosis.[68] It is probably the treatment of choice for hypercalcemia in children with non-Hodgkin's lymphoma and bony metastases.

4. *Calcitonin.* A dose of 2.0–8.0 MRC units/kg (salmon or porcine) produces reliable but short-lived hypocalcemia, both by reducing bone resorption and by enhancing calcium excretion.[97] Calcitonin also inhibits tubular reabsorption of calcium, phosphorus, and sodium and is also of value in children with hypercalcemia.[50]

HYPERPHOSPHATEMIA AND HYPOCALCEMIA

Hyperphosphatemia is well documented in patients with non-Hodgkin's lymphoma. It is particularly noted as a complication of the early treatment of disseminated Burkitt's lymphoma, which has a very high rate of cell proliferation, and is often extremely sensitive to chemotherapy.[5,98,99] Hyperphosphatemia has also been observed in acute lymphoblastic leukemia.[58,59] The presumed mechanism is the release of large amounts of phosphate ions from lysis of malignant lymphoid cells whose organic and inorganic phosphorus content is many times greater than that of normal lymphocytes.[100] Hyperphosphatemia has little direct toxicity[50] but it frequently produces hypocalcemia, presumably by calcium precipitation and diminished bone resorption.[91,101]

Other metabolic upsets frequently complicate the picture, including hyperkalemia,[56] lactic acidemia[102] and uric acid nephropathy, which lead to progressive renal insufficiency. This spectrum of coexisting metabolic disturbances has been aptly referred to as the *acute tumor lysis syndrome*.[5] Possible consequences of hyperphosphatemia and hypocalcemia include acute cardiac arrhythmias, neuromuscular irritability with carpopedal spasm, seizures, and ectopic calcifications in the kidneys leading to irreversible nephrocalcinosis. Successful management may require correction and maintenance of hydration with isotonic fluids, oral aluminum hydroxide, and intravenous calcium gluconate. Hemodialysis is sometimes needed.

HYPERKALEMIA

Hyperkalemia is seen in the same clinical setting as hyperphosphatemia. Presumably, hyperkalemia has a similar etiology, that is, the release of large quantities of potassium ions from rapid lysis of tumor cells during induction chemotherapy for lymphoma and acute leukemia.[56,103,104] There is a significant risk of sudden death from ventricular arrhythmias, particularly in the presence of renal insufficiency, acidemia, and hypocalcemia. Treatment consists of giving a sodium phase ion exchange (such as resin sodium polystyrene sulphonate at a dose of 0.5–1.0 g/kg/day in divided doses) or administering glucose and insulin infusions (consisting of 2.0 g/kg of dextrose and 1.0–2.0 units/kg of soluble insulin). If these treatments do not rapidly control the hyperkalemia, hemodialysis may be indicated.

LACTIC ACIDEMIA

In malignant disease, lactic acidemia may result from situations associated with severe hypoxemia, such as shock, sepsis, or pulmonary edema.[105] In leukemia and lymphoma, excessive anerobic glycolysis by tumor cells in the absence of systemic hypoxia may also cause this problem.[106] Lactic acid, produced by anerobic metabolism of glucose, is normally metabolized by the liver to carbon dioxide and water or stored as glycogen. Lactate production by lymphoma or leukemia cells may exceed the liver's capacity for lactate disposal, particularly if there is hepatic involvement by tumor.[102,107] Hyperkalemia, hyperuricemia, and other metabolic disturbances may coexist. Symptoms include generalized weakness, anorexia, and vomiting. Correction of acidosis depends upon effective treatment of the underlying neoplasm. However, initial therapy with intravenous sodium bicarbonate (at a dose of 0.5–2.0 mEq/kg/h) may be needed, aiming to limit rather than to completely correct the acidosis because of the risk of excessive sodium and fluid retention.

Because of the severity of the above metabolic complications, it is important to identify patients with non-Hodgkin's lymphomas who are at high risk of these complications at the time of presentation. These are children who have widespread disease at diagnosis, particularly those in whom there is bone, bone marrow, or renal involvement.[50] Particular attention should be paid to correcting any initial metabolic problems, monitoring renal and cardiac function, and maintaining good fluid and electrolyte balance. If the clinical situation allows, more gradual introduction of chemotherapy for the primary tumor should be tried. This approach will avoid some of these metabolic problems without reducing the likelihood of achieving complete remission.

SUMMARY

There are numerous well-recognized hazards that complicate the initial presentation and early treatment of non-Hodgkin's lymphoma (NHL) in children. This chapter reviews two groups of these disorders: (1) local mass effects of the tumor and (2) metabolic complications of the disease and its treatment. Mass effects include visual impairment from orbital involvement, respiratory obstruction from cervical or mediastinal nodal involvement or laryngeal infiltration, acute abdominal symptoms from extensive bowel and/or retroperitoneal nodal disease, and CNS complications produced by direct intracranial or paraspinal deposits. Principles of treatment include: rapid and accurate localization of tumor masses and the immediate institution of combined chemotherapy and radiotherapy with or without decompressive surgery.

Metabolic effects of NHL may occur singly or in combination. They result from the presence of extensive tumor spread, often exacerbated by therapy that produces rapid lysis of cancer cells. Metabolic complications include hyperuricemia, xanthinuria, hypercalcemia, hyperphosphatemia with hypocalcemia, hyperkalemia, and lactic acidemia. Children at particular risk of these disturbances must be identified at the time of presentation. Patients at high risk of metabolic complications include those with widespread disease involving the bones, bone marrow, and/or the kidneys.

Important measures to be taken are the maintenance of good fluid and electrolyte balance, monitoring of cardiac and renal function, and, as far as possible, correction of initial metabolic problems before initiating intensive anticancer therapy. Management of individual metabolic complications are also discussed.

References

1. Murphy SB: Management of childhood non-Hodgkin's lymphoma. *Cancer Treat Rep 61:1161–1173, 1977.*
2. Toledano SR, Meadows AT: Chapter 4, this volume.
3. Mott M: Chapter 5, this volume.
4. Timothy A, Freeman J: Chapter 6, this volume.
5. Ziegler J: Chapter 9, this volume.

6. Wollner N, Burchenal JH, Lieberman PH, *et al*: Non-Hodgkin's lymphoma in children. *Med Pediatr Oncol 1:235–263, 1975.*
7. Traggis DT, Jaffe N, Vawter G, *et al*: Non-Hodgkin's lymphoma of the head and neck in childhood. *J Pediatr 87:933–936, 1975.*
8. Jaffe BF, Jaffe N: Head and neck tumors in children. *Pediatrics 51:731–740, 1973.*
9. Kleener J: Lymphoma and other lymphoid lesions of the orbit. *Acta Ophthalmol 55:549–560, 1977.*
10. Lehrer S, Roswit B: Primary malignant lymphoma of the paranasal sinuses. *Ann Otol 87:81–84, 1978.*
11. Podoshin L, Talmon Y, Fraclis M: Malignant lymphoma of the maxillary sinus. *J Laryngol Otol 92:613–618, 1978.*
12. Shanmugham MS: Malignant lymphoma of the faucial tonsil. *J Laryngol Otol 92:357–324, 1978.*
13. Cohen SR, Landing BH, Byrne WJ, *et al*: Primary lymphosarcoma of the larynx in a child. *Ann Otol, Rhinol Laryngol 87:20–24, 1978.*
14. Wollner N, Burchenal JH, Lieberman PH, *et al*: Non-Hodgkin's lymphoma in children. *Cancer 37:123–134, 1976.*
15. D'Angio GJ, Mitus A, Evans AE: The superior mediastinal syndrome in children with cancer. *Am J Roentgenol 93:537–544, 1965.*
16. Elder JS, Touloukian RJ: Surgical diagnosis of mediastinal lymphoma of childhood. *Arch Surg 114:54–58, 1979.*
17. Lokich, JJ, Goodman R: Superior vena cava syndrome. *JAMA 231:58–61, 1975.*
18. Davenport D, Ferree C, Blake D, *et al*: Response of superior vena cava syndrome to radiation therapy. *Cancer 38:1577–1580, 1976.*
19. Bagby GC, Goldman RD, Newman HC, *et al*: Acute myocardial infarction due to childhood lymphoma. *N Engl J Med 287:338–340, 1972.*
20. Zea JM, Exelby PR, Wollner N: Abdominal non-Hodgkin's lymphoma in childhood. *J Pediatr Surg 11:363–369, 1976.*
21. Wayne ER, Campbell JB, Kosloske AM, *et al*: Intussusception in the older child; suspect lymphoma. *J Pediatr Surg 12:789–794, 1976.*
22. Jenkin RDT, Sonley MJ, Stephens MCA, *et al*: Primary gastrointestinal tract lymphoma in childhood. *Radiology 92:763–767, 1969.*
23. Jones SF, Tobias DA, Waldman RS: Computed tomographic scanning in patients with lymphoma. *Cancer 41:480–486, 1978.*
24. Cotman WE, Bloomfield CD, Amplatz K, *et al*: Lymphography as a guide during laparotomy in Hodgkin's and non-Hodgkin's lymphomas. *Acta Radiol Ther Phys Biol 16:295–304, 1977.*
25. Anderson T, Bender RA, Rosenoff SH, *et al*: Peritoneoscopy; a technique to evaluate therapeutic efficacy in non-Hodgkin's lymphoma patients. *Cancer Treat Rep 61:1017–1022, 1977.*
26. Carabell SC, Cassady JR, Weinstein HJ, *et al*: The rate of radiation therapy in the treatment of pediatric non-Hodgkin's lymphomas. *Cancer 42:2193, 2205, 1978.*
27. Murphy SB: Childhood non-Hodgkin's lymphoma. *N Engl J Med 299:1446–1448, 1978.*
28. Hutter JJ, Favara BE, Nelson M, *et al*: Non-Hodgkin's lymphoma in children; correlation of CNS disease with initial presentation. *Cancer 36:2132–2137, 1975.*
29. Willoughby MLN: Chapter 8, this volume.
30. Jenkin RDT: Radiation in the treatment of non-Hodgkin's lymphoma in children *Semin Oncol 4:311–315, 1977.*
31. Skarin AT, Tuckerman KS, Pitman SW, *et al*: High-dose methotrexate with folinic acid in the treatment of advanced non-Hodgkin's lymphoma including CNS development. *Blood 50:1039–1047, 1977.*
32. Brecher ML, Sinks LF, Thomas RRM, *et al*: Non-Hodgkin's lymphoma in children. *Cancer 41:1997–2001, 1978.*
33. Sullivan MP, Butler JJ: Non-Hodgkin's lymphoma of childhood, in Sutow WW, Vietti TJ, Fernbach DJ (eds): *Clinical Pediatric Oncology,* C. V. Mosby, St. Louis, 1977.

34. Sahn EE, Robinson WA: Spinal cord compression in lymphomas. *Am J Med Sci 276:93–98, 1978.*
35. Baten M, Vannucci RC: Intraspinal metastatic disease in childhood cancer. *J Pediatr 90:207–212, 1977.*
36. Tefft M, Mitus A, Schulz MD: Initial high dose irradiation for metastases causing spinal cord compression in children. *Am J Roentgenol 106:385–393, 1969.*
37. Friedman M, Kim T, Panahon AM: Spinal cord compression in malignant lymphoma. *Cancer 37:1485–1491, 1976.*
38. Khan FR, Glicksman AS, Chu FCH, *et al*: Treatment by radiotherapy of spinal cord compression due to extradural metastases. *Radiology 89:495–500, 1967.*
39. Kanfer A, Vandewalle A, Morel-Maroger L, *et al*: Acute renal insufficiency due to lymphomatous infiltration of the kidneys. *Cancer 38:2588–2592, 1976.*
40. Talbot J: Gout and blood dyscrasias. *Medicine 38:173–205, 1959.*
41. Weisberger A, Persky L: Renal calculi and uremia as complications of lymphoma. *Am J Med Sci 225:669–673, 1953.*
42. Greenbaum D, Stone M: Dangers of uric acid excretion during treatment of leukemia and lymphosarcoma. *Lancet 1:73–75, 1959.*
43. Frei E, Bentzel C, Rieselbach R, *et al*: Renal complications of neoplastic disease. *J Chron Dis 16:757–776, 1963.*
44. Pochedly C: Hyperuricemia in leukemia and lymphoma. I. Clinical findings and pathophysiology. *New York State J Med 73:1085–1092, 1973.*
45. Howard N: Acute renal failure in leukemia and lymphoma. *Br J Radiol 39:618–619, 1966.*
46. Yolken RN, Miller DR: Hyperuricemia and renal failure; presenting manifestations of occult hematologic malignancies. *J Pediatr 89:775–777, 1976.*
47. Krakoff IH, Murphy ML: Hyperuricemia in neoplastic disease in children; prevention with allopurinol, a xanthine oxidase inhibitor. *Pediatrics 41:52–56, 1968.*
48. Perry MC, Hoagland HC, Wagoner RD: Uric acid nephropathy. *JAMA 236:961–962, 1976.*
49. Kjellstrand CM, Campbell DC, Von Hartitzoh B, *et al*: Hyperuricemic acute renal failure. *Arch Intern Med 133:349–359, 1974.*
50. Lynch RE, Kjellstrand CM, Coccia PF: Renal and metabolic complications of childhood non-Hodgkin's lymphoma. *Semin Oncol 4:325–332, 1977.*
51. Whitaker JA, Shaheedy M, Baum J, *et al*: Gout in childhood leukemia. *J Pediatr 63:961–966, 1963.*
52. Kanwar YS, Manaligod JR: Leukemic urate nephropathy. *Arch Pathol 99:467–472, 1975.*
53. Rastegar A, Thier SO: The physiologic approach to hyperuricemia. *N Engl J Med 286:470–476, 1972.*
54. Klinenberg JR, Govnick HD, Dornfield L: Renal function abnormalities in patients with asymptomatic hyperuricemia. *Arthr Rheum 18(suppl):725–730, 1975.*
55. Primikirios N, Stutzman L, Sandberg A: Uric acid excretion in patients with malignant lymphoma. *Blood 17:701–718, 1961.*
56. Arsenau J, Bagley CM, Anderson T, *et al*: Hyperkalemia, a sequel to chemotherapy of Burkitt's lymphoma. *Lancet 1:10–14, 1973.*
57. Sinks LF, Newton WA, Nagi NA, *et al*: A syndrome associated with extreme hyperuricemia in leukemia. *J Pediatr 68:578–588, 1966.*
58. Zusman J, Brown DM, Nesbit ME: Hyperphosphatemia, hyperphosphaturia and hypocalcemia in acute lymphoblastic leukemia. *N Engl J Med 289:1335–1340, 1973.*
59. Jaffe N, Kim BS, Vawter GF: Hypocalcemia; a complication of childhood leukemia. *Cancer 29:392–398, 1972.*
60. Herrington RT, Fallon HJ: Uric acid nephropathy in leukemia. *N Engl J Med 266:934–935, 1962.*
61. Rundles RW, Wyngaarden JB, Hitchings GH, *et al*: Effects of xanthine oxidase inhibitor on thiopurine metabolism, hyperuricemia and gout. *Trans Assoc Am Physician 76:126–140, 1963.*

62. Barry KG, Hunter RN, Davis TE, *et al*: Acute uric acid nephropathy. *Arch Intern Med 111:452–459, 1963.*
63. Deger GE, Wagoner RD: Peritoneal dialysis in acute uric acid nephropathy. *Mayo Clin Proc 47:189–192, 1977.*
64. Band PR, Silverberg DS, Henderson JE, *et al*: Xanthine nephropathy in a patient with lymphosarcoma treated with allopurinol. *N Engl J Med 283:354–357, 1970.*
65. Ablin A, Stephens BG, Hiratat J, *et al*: Nephropathy, xanthinuria and orotic aciduria complicating Burkitt's lymphoma treated with chemotherapy and allopurinol. *Metabolism 21:771–778, 1972.*
66. Fox FM, Royse-Smith DR, O'Sullivan WJ: Orotidinuria induced by allopurinol. *Science 168:861–862, 1970.*
67. Lazor MZ, Rosenberg LE: Mechanism of adrenal steroid reversal of hypercalcemia in multiple myeloma. *N Engl J Med 270:749–755, 1964.*
68. Mazzaferri EL, O'Dorisio TM, Lobuglio AF: Treatment of hypercalcemia associated with malignancy. *Semin Oncol 5:141–153, 1978.*
69. Moses AM, Spencer H: Hypercalcemia in patients with malignant lymphoma. *Ann Intern Med 59:531–536, 1963.*
70. Canellos GP: Hypercalcemia in malignant lymphoma and leukemia. *Ann New York Acad Sci 230:240–246, 1974.*
71. Walker IR: Lymphoma with hypercalcemia. *Canad Med Assoc J 111:928–930, 1974.*
72. Stapleton FB, Lukert BP, Linshaw MA: Treatment of hypercalcemia associated with osseous metastases. *J Pediatr 89:1029–1030, 1976.*
73. Spiegel A, Greene M, Magrath I, *et al*: Hypercalcemia with suppressed parathyroid hormone in Burkitt's lymphoma. *Am J Med 64:691–695, 1978.*
74. Muggia FM, Heinemann MO: Hypercalcemia associated with neoplastic disease. *Ann Intern Med 73:281–290, 1970.*
75. Besarab A, Caro JF: Mechanisms of hypercalcemia in malignancy. *Cancer 41:2276–2285, 1978.*
76. Singer FR, Powell D, Minkin C, *et al*: Hypercalcemia in reticulum cell sarcoma without hyperparathyroidism or skeletal metastases. *Ann Intern Med 78:365–369, 1973.*
77. Sherwood LM, O'Riordan JLH, Aurbach GD, *et al*: Production of parathyroid hormone by nonparathyroid tumors. *J Clin Exp Med 27:140–146, 1967.*
78. Benson RC, Riggs BL, Pickard M: Immunoreactive forms of circulating parathormone in primary and ectopic hyperparathyroidism. *J Clin Invest 54:175–181, 1974.*
79. Tashjian AH: Role of prostaglandins in the production of hypercalcemia by tumors. *Cancer Res 38:4138–4141, 1978.*
80. Seyberth HW, Segre GV, Morgan JL, *et al*: Prostaglandins as mediators of hypercalcemia associated with certain types of cancer. *N Engl J Med 293:1278–1283, 1975.*
81. Mundy GR, Luben RA, Raisz LG, *et al*: Bone resorbing activity in supernatants from lymphoid cell lines. *N Engl J Med 290:867–871, 1974.*
82. Rasmussen H, Bordier P, Kurokawa K, *et al*: Hormonal control of skeletal and mineral homeostasis. *Am J Med 56:751–758, 1974.*
83. Riggs BL, Arnaud CD, Reynolds JC, *et al*: Immunologic differentiation of primary hyperparathyroidism due to non-parathyroid cancer. *J Clin Invest 50:2079–2083, 1971.*
84. Lokich J, Shevitz F: Hypercalcemia in malignant lymphoma; a case in a patient after parathyroidectomy. *JAMA 242:66–67, 1979.*
85. Mundy GR, Raisz LG, Cooper RA, *et al*: Evidence for the secretion of an osteoclast stimulating factor in myeloma. *N Engl J Med 291:1041–1046, 1974.*
86. Luben RA, Mundy, GR, Trummell CL, *et al*: Partial purification of osteoclast activating factor from phytohemaglutinin in stimulated human leukocytes. *J Clin Invest 53:1473–1480, 1974.*
87. Dudley FJ, Blackburn CRB: Extraskeletal calcification complicating oral neutral phosphate therapy. *Lancet 2:628–630, 1970.*
88. Goldsmith RD: Differential diagnosis of hypercalcemia. *N Engl J Med 274:674–677, 1966.*

89. Massry SG, Friedler RM, Coburn JW: Excretion of phosphate and calcium; physiology of their renal handling and relation to clinical medicine. *Arch Intern Med 131:828–836, 1973.*
90. Suki WN, Yium JJ, Von Minden M, *et al*: Acute treatment of hypercalcemia with furosemide. *N Engl J Med 283:836–840, 1970.*
91. Strauch BS, Ball MF: Hemodialysis in the treatment of severe hypercalcemia. *JAMA 235:1347–1348, 1976.*
92. Fulmer DH, Dimich AB, Rothschild EO, *et al*: Arch Intern Med 129:923—930.
93. Shackney S, Hasson J: Precipitous fall in serum calcium, hypotension and acute renal failure after intravenous phosphate therapy for hypercalcemia. *Ann Intern Med 66:906–916, 1967.*
94. Edwards CRW, Besser GM: Mithramycin treatment of malignant hypercalcemia. *Br Med J 3:167–168, 1968.*
95. Robins PR, Jowsey J: Effect of mithramycin on normal and abnormal bone turnover. *J Lab Clin Med 82:576–586, 1973.*
96. Slayton RE, Shnider B, Elias E, *et al*: New approach to the treatment of hypercalcemia. *Clin Pharmacol Ther 12:833–837, 1971.*
97. Vaughn CB, Vaitkevicius K: The effects of calcitonin in hypercalcemia in patients with malignancy. *Cancer 34:1268–1271, 1974.*
98. Brereton HD, Anderson T, Johnson RE, *et al*: Hyperphosphatemia and hypocalcemia in Burkitt's lymphoma. *Arch Intern Med 135:307–309, 1975.*
99. Cadman EC, Lundberg WB, Bertino JR: Hyperphosphatemia and hypocalcemia accompanying rapid cell lysis in a patient with Burkitt's lymphoma and Burkitt cell leukemia. *Am J Med 62:283–290, 1977.*
100. Rigas DA, Duerst ML, Jump ME, *et al*: The nucleic acids and other phosphorus compounds of human leukemic leucocytes; relation to cell maturity. *J Lab Clin Med 48:356–378, 1956.*
101. Hebert LA, Lemann J, Petersen JR, *et al*: Studies of the mechanism by which phosphate infusion lowers serum calcium concentration. *J Clin Invest 45:1886–1894, 1966.*
102. Block JB, Bronson WR, Bell WR: Metabolic abnormalities of lactic acid in Burkitt-type lymphoma with malignant effusions. *Ann Intern Med 64:101–108, 1966.*
103. Muggia FM: Hyperkalemia and chemotherapy. *Lancet 1:602–603, 1973.*
104. Fennelly JJ, Smyth H, Muldowney FP: Extreme hyperkalemia due to rapid lysis of leukemic cells. *Lancet 1:27, 1974.*
105. Oliva BP: Lactic acidosis. *Am J Med 48:209–225, 1970.*
106. Field M, Block JB, Levin R, *et al*: Significance of blood lactate elevations among patients with acute leukemia and other neoplastic proliferative disorders. *Am J Med 40:528–547, 1966.*
107. Mintz U, Sweet DL, Bitran JD, *et al*: Lactic acidosis and diffuse histiocytic lymphoma. *Am J Hematol 4:359–365, 1978.*

CHAPTER EIGHT

Burkitt's Lymphoma

JOHN L. ZIEGLER, MD

BURKITT'S LYMPHOMA IS A distinct histopathological entity within the spectrum of the malignant lymphomas.[1,2] Burkitt's lymphoma is endemic in tropical Africa and New Guinea, where it has been associated with chronic malaria[3] and the Epstein-Barr virus (EBV)[4]; it also occurs sporadically world-wide. Though the true incidence is not known, between 200 and 300 cases are diagnosed annually in the U.S.A.[5] Study of Burkitt's lymphoma provides insights into neoplasia in general because of its association with the EB virus, because of its unusual immunologic and biologic features, and because of its remarkable responses to therapy. This chapter will review each of these topics, highlighting current advances in the biology and treatment of this unusual lymphoma.

THE NEOPLASTIC CELL OF BURKITT'S LYMPHOMA

Surface marker studies have confirmed the B-cell nature of Burkitt's lymphoma by the presence of surface immunoglobulin and the presence of complement receptor and Fc receptors. These findings are consistent with its follicular pattern of origin and spread.[2] Burkitt's lymphoma is monoclonal in origin, as demonstrated by genetic marker studies.[6] Some tumors exhibit an 8-14q chromosomal translocation.[7] Kinetic studies on Burkitt's lymphoma cells reveal a doubling time of 24 h, with a growth fraction approaching 100%.[8] There is a high rate of spontaneous cell death. In endemic cases, Burkitt's lymphoma cells contain the EB virus genome in the DNA, and such cells express a variety of EB viral-associated antigens which elicit antibody and cell-mediated responses.[9]

Clinical Oncology Program, Division of Cancer Treatment, National Cancer Institute, Bethesda, MD 20014

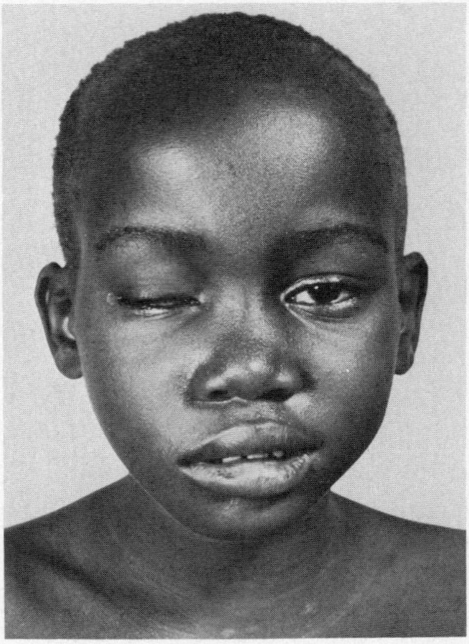

FIG. 1. This nine-year-old girl presented with jaw and ovarian tumors which regressed promptly following treatment with cyclophosphamide. Ten weeks later, she experienced the onset of diplopia. Within several days third and seventh cranial nerve palsies were evident on the right. Burkitt lymphoma cells were found in the cerebrospinal fluid.

ETIOLOGY

Following the original description of Burkitt's lymphoma, it was recognized that climatic determinants, defined by temperature, rainful, and altitude, created a "lymphoma belt" through tropical Africa, and suggested a vectored virus as a cause. It was recognized subsequently that chronic, holoendemic malaria accounted for the geographic distribution.[10] Etiologic studies also led to the discovery of the EB virus in cultured Burkitt's lymphoma cells. This ubiquitous virus was found to infect over 80% of Ugandan children before the age of 10 years. A prospective sero-epidemiologic survey revealed that an acute infection with EB virus is not the proximate "cause" of Burkitt's lymphoma, although high titers of anti-EB viral antibodies were identified up to three years prior to the development of the tumor.[11] A full discussion of the roles of malaria, EB virus, and other possible etiologic cofactors is beyond the scope of this chapter, but excellent reviews can be found.[4,11-13]

CLINICAL FEATURES

In Africa, the mean age of onset is 7 years, with a range of 2 to 16 years; in the U.S.A., the mean age is 11 years with a range of 2 to 45 years. In Africa, most

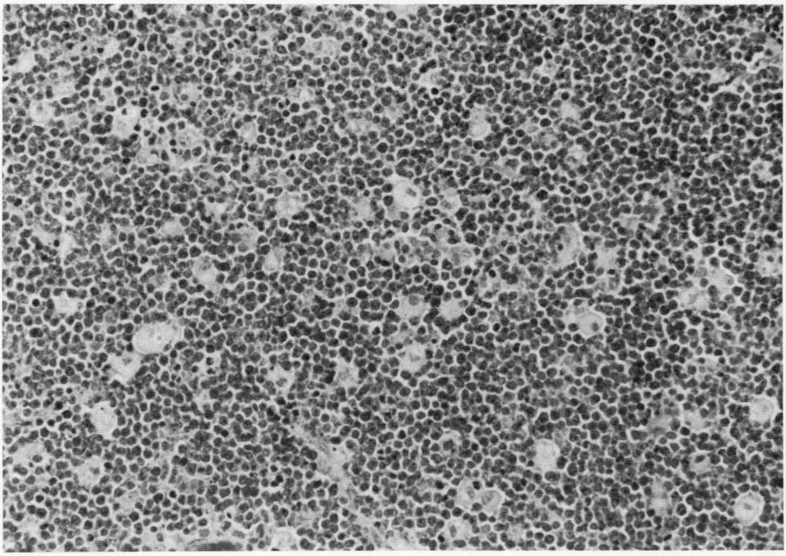

FIG. 2. Typical histologic features of Burkitt's lymphoma. Note the uniformity of cell size and shape. Macrophages interspersed among malignant lymphoblasts give a "starry sky" pattern. (H&E stain, reduced from ×100).

tumors localize to the jaws and retroperitoneal space; bilateral involvement of kidneys and ovaries is common, and paraspinal tumors account for 15% of presentations. Tumor infiltration of lymphoreticular tissue (such as lymph nodes, liver, spleen, and bone marrow) is uncommon. In the U.S.A., and in other nonendemic areas, the presenting sites of involvement are predominantly lymphoid. The most common site is the gastrointestinal tract in the ileocecal region. Next in frequency is cervical lymphadenopathy and bone marrow involvement. More rarely, the clinician will encounter the "typical" tumor distribution seen in Africa, in which the jaws, ovaries, and paraspinal areas are involved. Other than these clinical differences, plus the strong association with EB virus in endemic areas, patients with Burkitt's lymphoma have similar clinical behavior and responses to treatment wherever they are encountered.[14]

Spread to the central nervous system (CNS), either on initial presentation or as a manifestation of relapse, is a common event.[15,16] This complication is heralded most frequently by the rapid development of single or multiple cranial nerve palsies, due to direct infiltration of the nerve by tumor. A clinical example is shown in Fig. 1. Malignant cells are seen in the cerebrospinal fluid.[17] The pathogenesis of CNS spread is still uncertain. Factors that carry increased risk of CNS involvement include bone marrow involvement, tumors in the head and neck, paraspinal tumors, and advanced clinical stage. These factors suggest that tumor may spread in contiguity to the CNS either directly or via cranial or spinal nerves, or may be

TABLE 1
Staging of Burkitt's Lymphoma in Africa[23]

Stage	Site of involvement
A	Solitary extraabdominal site
AR	Resected intraabdominal tumor
B	Multiple extraabdominal sites
C	Intraabdominal tumor with or without facial tumors
D	Intraabdominal tumors (stage C) with sites of tumor other than facial

blood-borne. In either case, tumor in the CNS necessitates both preventive and therapeutic "sanctuary" therapy.

CLINICAL EVALUATION

Particular urgency is required in the diagnosis, evaluation, and initial management of patients with Burkitt's lymphoma. The diagnosis can be readily established cytologically by fine needle aspiration of the tumor, examination of malignant effusion, or a tumor imprint. This can be accomplished within minutes of obtaining tumor tissue.[17] Histologic diagnosis may present difficulty in interpretation and classification because of fixation artifacts. The diagnosis should be confirmed by a hematologist or pathologist experienced in the identification of malignant lymphomas. The characteristic histologic features are shown in Fig. 2.

Clinical evaluation must seek major sites of tumor involvement, but rigorous identification of every tumor deposit is unnecessary since systemic chemotherapy is the treatment of choice. Among the clinical and laboratory detection methods mentioned elsewhere in this book, the determination of bone marrow and CNS involvement and a careful assessment of renal function are particularly important. Diffuse bone marrow invasion indicates that the patient may have profound and prolonged pancytopenia after chemotherapy, often necessitating vigorous hematologic support. Rarely "Burkitt's leukemia" will be the dominant presenting feature, although a careful search may disclose solid tumor deposits.[18] CNS involvement, with the exception of paraplegia, is usually occult on admission, and is manifested only by the presence of malignant cells in the CSF. Rarely, Burkitt's lymphoma appears as a solid intracranial tumor.[19] ^{67}Gallium scintigraphy and determination of serum lactic dehydrogenase levels are the most useful supplements to the physical examination in detecting the presence of Burkitt's lymphoma and in monitoring patients during remission.[20-22]

Childhood lymphoma does not lend itself to systematic clinical and pathologic staging, such as that currently recommended in Hodgkin's disease and adult lymphomas. Because Burkitt's lymphoma occurs in varied anatomic sites, and size of the tumor appears to be prognostically more important than location, attempts at

TABLE 2
Management of Acute Tumor Lysis Syndrome

Problem	Possible causes	Assessment	Corrective action
Pretreatment			
Azotemia	Hyperuricemia, obstruction, intrarenal tumor	BUN, creatinine, uric acid, serum urine electrolytes, Ca, PO_4, IVP, renal scan. Monitor electrolytes 8 hourly	Hydration, lasix; lower urate levels with allopurinol and urine alkalinization; dialysis
Dehydration	Poor intake, fever, third space (ascites)	Clinical; urinalysis, blood volume, CVP. Monitor CVP, cardiac status	Intravenous hydration with 5% dextrose in ¼ normal saline
Acidosis	Hyperlactacidemia, hypoventilation (pleural effusion, ascites)	Clinical; serum and urine pH, lactate, pyruvate, electrolytes	Intravenous bicarbonate; titrate urine to pH 6.5-7
Post treatment (acute tumor lysis)			
Azotemia	Hyperuricemia	Serum urate, urinalysis	Continued hydration, allopurinol, alkalinization; dialysis
Hyperphosphatemia	Poor renal excretion of phosphate	Serum, urine phosphate	Hydration; lower urine pH; dialysis
Hypocalcemia	Hyperphosphatemia	Clinical; ECG Serum Ca, PO_4	Slow infusion of Ca gluconate if symptomatic; lower serum phosphate
Hyperkalemia	Renal failure, acidosis	Serum electrolytes	Severe: Glucose and insulin infusion, dialysis Moderate: Hydrate, correct acidosis, chelating agent

clinical staging have varied considerably. In Africa, larger patient numbers permit more staging strata, which define a gradient of increasing tumor burden. A system in current use is shown in Table 1.[23] In the U.S.A. and elsewhere, only two stages (small tumors vs. large tumors) thus far have been shown to have prognostic import.[14]

ACUTE TUMOR LYSIS SYNDROME

Patients with large tumors may have impaired renal function as manifested by azotemia, lowered glomerular filtration rate, and oliguria. These patients are at high risk of developing the acute tumor lysis syndrome during initiation of chemotherapy.[24] Predisposing factors include a large tumor burden, elevated uric acid, elevated lactic acid, dehydration, obstructive uropathy, and kidney involvement by tumor. Urate nephropathy, resulting from tumor necrosis and purine catabolism, is usually the primary cause of impaired renal function.

This complication requires immediate correction with hydration, vigorous diuresis, and alkalinization with bicarbonate prior to and during the initiation of chemotherapy (Table 2). If the patient remains oliguric and urate levels are over 10 mg/dl despite these measures, hemodialysis (or peritoneal dialysis) is indicated. Corrective action is particularly critical if the tumor is very large, since clearance of tumor breakdown products during chemotherapy will depend on adequate renal function. Lactic acidosis, a consequence of a large, anaerobic, hypermetabolic tumor, and aggravated by hypoxemia, may complicate the acid-base stability, and contribute to urate nephropathy.[25] Vigorous alkalinization will also tend to reverse the metabolic acidosis.

Within the first 48 h of induction chemotherapy, further metabolic derangement can be anticipated. Acute tumor lysis leads to release of tumor intracellular contents, especially phosphate.[25] Under circumstances of normal renal function and high urine volume, urinary phosphate levels rise steeply, but serum phosphate will remain within the normal range. If azotemia and oliguria are present, serum phosphate may rise steeply, causing a compensatory drop in ionized calcium, leading to clinical tetany. Serum potassium may also rise as a consequence of tumor necrosis, but can be aggravated by metabolic acidosis, renal impairment, and dehydration.[26] Sudden cardiac arrest in patients with Burkitt's lymphoma following treatment has been attributed to lethal cardiac arrhythmias resulting from these electrolyte disturbances; that is, high potassium and low calcium.[25,26] Clinicians must anticipate the acute tumor lysis syndrome. It is very important to achieve metabolic stability and adequate renal function prior to therapy, and to provide close metabolic monitoring of high risk patients during the period of induction of chemotherapy.

SURGICAL TREATMENT

Surgery has an important place in the initial management of Burkitt's lymphoma. Although the value of surgery is not established by randomized clinical trial, all available evidence indicates that surgical reduction of tumor bulk improves prognosis. Both in endemic and nonendemic areas, surgical resection of greater than 90% of tumor more than doubles the duration of survival, independent of other prognostic factors such as age.[27] This observation has led to a stage designated AR, for *abdominal resection*, since this is the only anatomic site where resection of bulky tumor is feasible. Thus when the surgeon explores the abdomen of a patient with abdominal Burkitt's lympoma and decides that curative resection cannot be performed, he should attempt to reduce tumor burden as much as possible. Surgical reduction of tumor burden may include bowel and mesentery resection, nephrectomy, ovariectomy/hysterectomy, and other forms of extirpative surgery.

Obstructive complications resulting from rapid tumor growth may require urgent surgical intervention. Over half of the American patients presenting with Burkitt's lymphoma develop intraabdominal tumor, very often arising in Peyer's patches in the ileocecal area. Thus intussusception or acute bowel obstruction may result. When tumor is found, a bowel resection is usually performed, followed by end-to-end anastomosis. Occasionally, during treatment of lymphoma involving the bowel wall, perforation through a necrotic tumor nodule will occur, resulting in acute peritonitis and a surgical emergency. Finally, it must be remembered that even patients whose tumor has recurred may benefit from extensive surgical resection. Reduction of tumor bulk in this setting may still improve prognosis. The role of surgical reduction of residual tumor following chemotherapy has not been examined; since tumor tends to recur in sites of previous bulk disease, this approach bears further investigation.

RADIOTHERAPY

Early reports of the results of radiotherapy as a primary mode of treatment of Burkitt's lymphoma were disappointing. Subsequent experience revealed that hyperfractionated dose schedules were required to achieve complete responses.[28] This approach, while not yet employed widely by radiotherapists, is logical in view of the rapid proliferative rate of the tumor. Radiotherapy in conventional doses and fractions has been used in patients with localized, extraabdominal tumor deposits. Likewise, neuraxis irradiation has been employed in patients with CNS involvement, such as those with meningeal spread or paraspinal tumor. Since systemic chemotherapy is often used concomitantly, it is not possible to assess the effect of radiotherapy alone in these settings. Because the tumor is widespread, radiotherapy alone is never the treatment of choice, and should, if employed at all, be accompanied by systemic chemotherapy.

Two studies utilizing radiotherapy as part of the overall treatment strategy deserve mention. In one, 2100 rad was delivered to the whole abdomen in patients in remission who had presented initially with abdominal tumors. Radiotherapy was given after three courses of chemotherapy in an attempt to avert abdominal relapse. Of 23 patients so treated, 8 developed recurrent abdominal tumors.[14] In

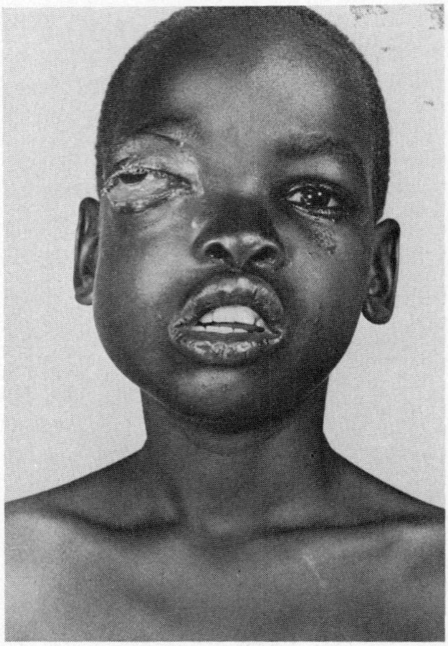

FIG. 3. Burkitt's lymphoma involves the right orbit and maxilla in this eleven-year-old boy.

another study, a dose of 2400 rad of craniospinal irradiation was given in a randomized study to a group of patients in complete remission, in an effort to prevent CNS recurrence. Of 11 patients so treated, meningeal relapse occurred in 6, as compared to 4 such relapses that occurred in 11 control patients.[29] Thus "prophylactic" radiotherapy following remission was not effective in averting relapse in either the abdomen or the CNS.

CHEMOTHERAPY

Burkitt's lymphoma is sensitive to a wide range of cytotoxic agents.[30] The dramatic tumor regression observed following chemotherapy is illustrated in Figs. 3 and 4. The most effective single agents are cyclophosphamide (Cytoxan), orthomelphalan, methotrexate, vincristine (Oncovin), and cytosine arabinoside (Cytosar). Active, but less effective, agents include adriamycin, nitrosoureas, 6-mercaptopurine (Purinethol), and prednisone. Several compounds are shown to be relatively inactive, including daunomycin (Daunorubicin), L-asparaginase, and bleomycin.

A number of principles of chemotherapeutic strategy for Burkitt's lymphoma have evolved during the past 15 years:

1. Therapy should be given in high dose, intermittent courses.
2. Combination chemotherapy is probably more effective than single agents.

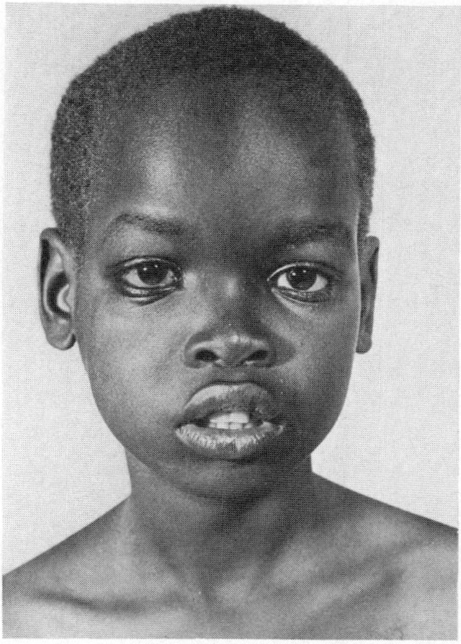

FIG. 4. Appearance of the same child in Fig. 3 after three courses of cyclophosphamide. All evidence of tumor has disappeared.

3. The role of maintenance therapy is unsettled, but relapse seldom occurs in patients with complete remission in excess of six months.
4. Prophylactic intrathecal chemotherapy, craniospinal irradiation, and nitrosourea therapy during induction do not appear to avert central nervous system relapse.
5. Reduction in tumor bulk by surgical resection prior to initial chemotherapy is beneficial.

Induction of remission should include intravenous cyclophosphamide in large, single doses (e.g., at least 40 mg/kg). The addition of vincristine, methotrexate, or cytosine arabinoside appears to increase the rate and durability of complete remissions.[31-33] The use of corticosteroids in Burkitt's lymphoma is controversial, since the tumor cells lack corticosteroid receptors in high concentration.[34] The addition of high-dose prednisolone to the combination of cyclophosphamide, vincristine, and methotrexate did not increase the complete response rate or remission duration in a sequential trial.[14] Two treatment regimens are shown in Table 3, and are code-named COM and COMP. At least three induction courses are recommended, and perhaps as many as six courses should be given if the initial tumor is large or extensive. Intervals between courses of treatment should be as short as possible, and should be dictated by the recovery of the white blood count to 4500/mm^3.[14]

TABLE 3
Two Treatment Regimens for Burkitt's Lymphoma[14]

Drug	Dose (mg/m^2)	Route	Schedule[a]
COM Regimen			
Cyclophosphamide	1000	IV	Day 1
Vincristine (Oncovin)	1.4	IV	Day 1
Methotrexate	15	IT	Days 1,4
Methotrexate	15	IV	Days 2,3
COMP Regimen[b]			
Cyclophosphamide	1000	IV	Day 1
Vincristine (Oncovin)	1.4	IV	Day 1
Methotrexate	12.5	IT	Days 2,5
Methotrexate	12.5	IV	Days 1,3,4
Prednisolone	1000	IV	Days 1-5

[a]Three chemotherapy courses are repeated at two week intervals (i.e., beginning on days 1, 15, and 27); courses are delayed until total leukocyte count is above $4500/mm^3$.

[b]Instead of a third induction course, patients receive cyclophosphamide, 1200 mg/m^2 intravenously on each of two successive days. Methotrexate, 12.5 mg/m^2, is given intrathecally (IT) on the first day of double-dose cyclophosphamide, followed by leucovorin rescue at a dose of 5.0 mg intramuscularly every six hours for four doses.

Note: Two weeks following the completion of chemotherapy, all patients with stages C, D, and AR receive 2100 rad whole abdominal radiation during a period of 18 elapsed days.

Treatment results using a variety of induction regimens are listed in Table 4. Variations in response rates, remission duration, and mortality are attributable to differences in referral patterns, diagnostic and staging criteria, trial design, definitions of response, and patient surveillance. In view of these many variables, the similarity of the clinical courses in African and American patients is indeed remarkable.

RELAPSE AND TREATMENT STRATEGY

While no "standard" treatment regimen can be recommended, current therapeutic strategy is aimed at (1) avoidance of early complications, (2) prevention of relapse, (3) prophylaxis of meningeal involvement, and (4) anticipation of "salvage" therapy for relapse. Averting early complications involves awareness of the acute tumor lysis syndrome and its management, and has been dealt with above.

Successful prevention of tumor relapse involves the identification of prognostic factors that indicate increased risk of relapse. Thus far, these unfavorable prognostic factors are tumor stage (high risk for stages C and D) and age (over 13 years).[14] For these patients, a more aggressive treatment approach should be sought. Such a strategy might include intensive consolidation chemotherapy, aggressive surgical excision of tumor (either before or after induction chemotherapy), and irradiation

TABLE 4
Treatment Results in Burkitt's Lymphoma in Africa and the U.S.A.

Regimen	Number evaluable	Complete response (CR)	Partial response	Relapse/CR	Reference
Africa					
CTX	18	15 (83%)	3	7/15 (47%)	31
	42	34 (81%)	8	21/34 (62%)	32
	79	74 (94%)	5	46/74 (62%)	30
COM	19	16 (84%)	3	10/16 (32%)	31
CVA	31	29 (99%)	2	9/29 (31%)	32
TRIKE	22	21 (95%)	1	12/21 (57%)	33
U.S.A.					
COM	27	27 (100%)	0	13/27 (48%)	14
COMP	23	21 (92%)	2	9/21 (43%)	14

Abbreviations: CTX = cyclophosphamide; COM = cyclophosphamide, vincristine (Oncovin), and methotrexate; CVA = cyclophosphamide, vincristine, and arabinosyl cytosine; TRIKE = cyclophosphamide alternating with vincristine and methotrexate, and arabinosyl cytosine; COMP = COM plus prednisolone (see Table 2).

(in hyperfractionated doses) of tumor bulk. Such approaches derive from clinical experience that (1) a large tumor burden is indicative of a poor prognosis, (2) an apparent dose-response relationship exists with respect to alkylating agents,[30,35,36] (3) tumors tend to recur in sites of previous bulky disease,[37] and (4) cytokinetic theory implies that increasingly intensive therapy might be beneficial in responsive tumors.[38]

Successful prophylaxis of meningeal involvement has not been achieved. Intrathecal chemotherapy during induction, the addition of CCNU to the initial treatment regimen, and craniospinal irradiation have not succeeded in averting meningeal relapse in controlled trials.[17,29] Design of successful protocols for prophylactic CNS therapy is thwarted by our ignorance regarding the pathogenesis of CNS involvement. Patients at greatest risk of CNS involvement are those who present with tumor in proximity to the CNS (such as those with head and neck and paraspinal tumors) suggesting direct spread. Likewise, patients presenting with bone marrow involvement show high rates of CNS involvement, which implies hematogenous spread to the CNS.

Although prophylactic measures have been unsuccessful, appropriate treatment of overt meningeal disease may provide long-term disease control. The mainstay of such treatment is intrathecal chemotherapy. The regimen of choice is intrathecal cytosine arabinoside, 30 mg/m^2 given on days one and three, and methotrexate, 15 mg/m^2 given on day four. This regimen should be repeated every other week for two courses beyond normalization of the CSF. While not proven to be beneficial, cranial irradiation (2500 rad) can be given concomitantly. A substantial number of patients from both endemic and nonendemic areas are long survivors following intrathecal treatment for established meningeal involvement.

Relapse after remission in diffuse undifferentiated lymphomas of adults usually terminates in death after a rapid downhill course, which may be prolonged somewhat by brief, partial remissions. Rarely, if ever, can such patients achieve durable second remissions. Such is not the case, however, with Burkitt's lymphoma. In endemic regions, two distinct forms of relapse have been identified.[39,40] *Early* relapse, occurring within the first three months of therapy, probably represents regrowth of original tumor, with or without "sanctuary" spread to the CNS. Attempts at reinduction, except in those few cases where initial therapy was inadequate, are frustrated by the rapid development of drug resistance. The majority of these patients die within six months of relapse. *Late* relapse, on the other hand, develops after a three month interval, often appears in a previously uninvolved site, generally spares the CNS, and responds rapidly and completely to therapy with the same agents used initially. The pathogenesis of late relapse is unknown, but may represent tumor "reinduction," particularly in those rare instances where there was disease-free interval of many years prior to relapse. In nonendemic regions, *late* relapse is uncommon, but where it does occur, the clinical behavior is similar to cases described in Africa.[12] There is a suggestion, as yet unconfirmed, that this form of relapse is more common among patients whose tumors harbor the EB virus and who display high titers of antibody to early antigen, restricted type.[9]

This unusual relapse pattern provided stimulus for a study of immunotherapy in Burkitt's lymphoma.[41] While it is beyond the scope of this chapter to present the immunology of Burkitt's lymphoma, excellent reviews can be found.[4,10,11,13,41] It was reasoned that BCG might correct the general and tumor-directed anergy associated with a large tumor burden and early relapse. A controlled randomized trial addressed this question, and two conclusions were reached: (1) BCG accelerated recovery of delayed hypersensitivity following chemotherapy-induced remissions; and (2) despite improved immunologic status, the relapse frequency and duration of remission were unaltered by BCG.

Because of the potential for durable complete responses in patients with Burkitt's lymphoma in relapse, aggressive reinduction chemotherapy is mandatory. Determination of CNS and bone marrow involvement, even in the absence of clinical signs or symptoms, must be carried out. As recommended above, surgical reduction of tumor bulk should be attempted where possible. Induction chemotherapy, with all of the precautions for tumor lysis syndrome, should begin promptly once the diagnosis and relapse stage are determined and metabolic stability is achieved. Concomitantly, therapy of evident meningeal disease can commence; the intrathecal chemotherapy regimen outlined above, plus cranial radiation, is recommended. Failure to respond completely to reinduction therapy, which must contain high dose cyclophosphamide, indicates a poor prognosis. In this situation, "second line" agents invariably fail to achieve satisfactory disease control. In the setting of alkylating agent resistant relapse, patients rapidly develop widespread disease with malignant effusions, CNS involvement, and bone marrow involvement, and succumb within several weeks of relapse despite vigorous therapy.

Recently, a more aggressive attempt at the management of early relapse has yielded encouraging results.[35,42] A four-day induction regimen (BACT) consisting of BCNU, arabinosyl cytosine (Cytosar), cyclophosphamide, and thioguanine was used. In some cases chemotherapy was followed by infusion of autologous bone marrow, that is, bone marrow from the patient harvested and cryopreserved while the patient was in remission. This regimen was administered to 14 patients with Burkitt's lymphoma in relapse, who were refractory to standard reinduction therapy. Four patients with very large tumors died within one week; three had acute carditis attributed to therapy. Of the remaining 10, six had partial responses and four had complete responses. Three of the patients who had complete responses have enjoyed prolonged unmaintained remissions in excess of two years; the remaining seven patients relapsed and died. This encouraging result has prompted further efforts at modifying reinduction therapy to avoid cardiac complications and to improve hematologic supportive care in the form of stem cell replenishment. Consideration is being given to advancing such aggressive treatment to the initial induction regimen in patients at high risk of relapse, such as older patients and those with tumors in advanced stages.

SUMMARY

Burkitt's lymphoma is the fastest growing neoplasm in man. As such, early diagnosis, awareness of complications, and knowledge of therapeutic strategy are critical factors in achieving a successful outcome. Since the disease is curable in over 50% of patients, every therapeutic effort should be applied to this objective. Because of the aggressive nature of the disease, there is little time for demurring over the diagnosis or a leisurely staging process.

Finally, though the tumor is rare in the U.S.A., Burkitt's lymphoma continues to provide a useful clinical model for therapeutic strategy based on tumor kinetics. For example, aggressive management of drug-resistant relapse has yielded durable complete responses in clinical situations that were considered hopeless. Therapeutic principles derived from Burkitt's lymphoma should be successfully applied to other human neoplasms in developing drug regimens aimed at cure.

References

1. Berard C, O'Conor GT, Thomas LB, *et al*: Histopathological definitions of Burkitt's tumour. *Bull WHO 40:601–607, 1969.*
2. Mann RB, Jaffe ES, Braylan RC, *et al*: Non-endemic Burkitt's lymphoma. A B-cell tumor related to germinal centers. *New Engl J Med 295:685–691, 1976.*
3. Burkitt DP: Long-term remissions following one and two-dose chemotherapy for African lymphoma. *Cancer 20:756–759, 1967.*
4. Klein G: The Epstein-Barr virus and neoplasia. *New Engl J Med 293:1353–1357, 1975.*

5. Levine PH, Cho BS, Connelly RR, *et al*: The American Burkitt lymphoma registry — a progress report. *Ann Intern Med 83:31–36, 1975.*
6. Fialkow PJ, Klein E, Klein G, *et al*: Immunoglobulin and glucose-6-phosphate dehydrogenase as markers of cellular organ in Burkitt lymphoma. *J Exp Med 138:89–102, 1973.*
7. Zech L, Haglund U, Nilsson K, *et al*: Characteristic chromosomal abnormalities in biopsies and lymphoid cell lines from patients with Burkitt and non-Burkitt lymphomas. *Int J Cancer 17:47–56, 1976.*
8. Iversen O, Iversen U, Ziegler JL, et al: Cell kinetics in Burkitt's lymphoma. *Eur J Cancer 10:155–163, 1974.*
9. Nkrumah FK, Henle W, Henle G, *et al*: Burkitt's lymphoma. Its clinical course in relation to immunologic reactivities to Epstein-Barr virus and tumor-related antigens. *J Natl Cancer Inst 57:1051–1056, 1976.*
10. Burkitt DP: Etiology of Burkitt's lymphoma — an alternative hypothesis to a vectored virus. *J Natl Cancer Inst 42:19–28, 1969.*
11. De Thé G, Geser A, Day NE, *et al*: Epidemiological evidence for a causal relationship between Epstein-Barr virus and Burkitt's lymphoma from Ugandan prospective study. *Nature 274:756–761, 1978.*
12. Ziegler JL, Magrath IT, Gerber P, *et al*: Epstein-Barr virus and human malignancy. *Ann Intern Med 86:323–336, 1977.*
13. Ziegler JL, Andersson M, Klein G, *et al*: Detection of Epstein-Barr virus (EBV) DNA in American Burkitt's lymphoma. *Intl J Cancer 17:701–706, 1976.*
14. Ziegler JL: Treatment results of 54 American patients with Burkitt's lymphoma are similar to the African experience. *New Engl J Med 297:75–80, 1977.*
15. Nkrumah FK, Perkins IV: Neurological manifestations of Burkitt's lymphoma in Ghana. *Afr J Med Sci 4:209–214, 1973.*
16. Ziegler JL, Bluming AZ, Morrow RH, *et al*: Central nervous system involvement in Burkitt's lymphoma. *Blood 36:718–728, 1970.*
17. Ziegler JL, Bluming AZ: Intrathecal chemotherapy in Burkitt's lymphoma. *Br Med J 3:508–512, 1971.*
18. Stevens DA, O'Conor GT, Levine PH, *et al*: Acute leukemia with "Burkitt's lymphoma cells" and Burkitt's lymphoma. Simultaneous onset in American siblings: description of a new entity. *Ann Intern Med 76:967–973, 1972.*
19. Magrath IT, Mugerwa J, Bailey I, *et al*: Intracerebral Burkitt's lymphoma: Pathology, clinical features, and treatment. *Quart J Med 43:489–508, 1974.*
20. Arseneau JC, Canellos GP, Banks PM, *et al*: American Burkitt's lymphoma — a clinicopathologic study of 30 cases. I. Clinical factors relating to prolonged survival. *Am J Med 58:314–321, 1975.*
21. Richman SD, Appelbaum FR, Levenson SM, *et al*: ^{67}Ga radionuclide imaging in Burkitt's lymphoma. *Radiology 117:639–645, 1975.*
22. Ziegler JL, DeVita VT, Graw RG Jr, *et al*: Combined modality treatment of American Burkitt's lymphoma. *Cancer 38:2225–2231, 1976.*
23. Ziegler JL, Magrath IT: Burkitt's lymphoma, in Ioachim HL (ed): *Pathobiology Annual.* Appleton-Century Crofts, New York, 1974, pp. 129—142.
24. Cohen LF, Balow JE, Magrath IT, *et al*: Acute tumor lysis syndrome; a review of 37 patients with Burkitt's lymphoma. *Am J Med* (in press).
25. Brereton HD, Anderson T, Johnson RE, *et al*: Hyperphosphatemia and hypocalcemia in Burkitt lymphoma. *Arch Intern Med 135:307–309, 1975.*
26. Arseneau JC, Bagley CM, Anderson T, *et al*: Hyperkalemia, a sequel to chemotherapy of Burkitt's lymphoma. *Lancet 1:10–14, 1973.*
27. Magrath IT, Lwanga S, Carswell W, *et al*: Surgical reduction of tumour bulk in management of abdominal Burkitt's lymphoma. *Br Med J 2:308–312, 1974.*
28. Norin T, Clifford P, Einhorn J, *et al*: Conventional and superfractionated radiation therapy in Burkitt's lymphoma. *Acta Radiol 10:545–557, 1971.*

29. Olweny CLM, Atine I, Kaddu-Mukasa A, *et al*: Cerebrospinal irradiation of Burkitt's lymphoma: failure in preventing central nervous system relapse. *Acta Radiol 16:225–231, 1977.*
30. Ziegler JL: Chemotherapy of Burkitt's lymphoma. *Cancer 30:1534–1540, 1972.*
31. Olweny CLM, Katongole-Mbidde E, Kaddu-Mukasa A, *et al*: Treatment of Burkitt's lymphoma: Randomized clinical trial of single agent versus combination chemotherapy. *Int J Cancer 17:436–440, 1976.*
32. Nkrumah FK, Perkins IV, Biggar RJ: Combination chemotherapy in abdominal Burkitt's lymphoma. *Cancer 40:1410–1416, 1977.*
33. Ziegler JL, Bluming AZ, Carbone PP: Intensive chemotherapy in patients with generalized Burkitt's lymphoma. *Int J Cancer 10:254–261, 1972.*
34. Lippman ME, Yarbro JK, Leventhal BG: Glucocorticoid receptors in normal and leukemia human leukocytes, in Bell PA, Borthwick NM (eds): *Glucocorticoid Action and Leukemia*. AOA Publishers, Cardiff, 1978.
35. Appelbaum FR, Deisseroth AB, Graw RG, *et al*: Prolonged complete remission following high dose chemotherapy of Burkitt's lymphoma in relapse. *Cancer 41:1059–1063, 1978.*
36. Durodola JI: Burkitt's lymphoma in Ibadan. Response to various doses of cyclophosphamide and long-term survivors. *Eur J Cancer 12:425–432, 1976.*
37. Nkrumah FK, Perkins IV: Burkitt's lymphoma: a clinical study of 110 patients. *Cancer 37:671–676, 1976.*
38. Norton L, Simon RS: Tumor size, sensitivity to therapy, and the design of treatment schedules. *Cancer Treat Rep 61:1307–1317, 1977.*
39. Nkrumah FK, Perkins IV: Relapse in Burkitt's lymphoma. *Int J Cancer 17:445–460, 1976.*
40. Ziegler JL, Bluming AZ, Morrow RH *et al*: Relapse patterns in Burkitt's lymphoma. *Cancer Res 32:1267–1272, 1972.*
41. Magrath IT, Ziegler JL: Failure of BCG immunostimulation to affect the clinical course of Burkitt's lymphoma. *Br Med J 1:615–618, 1976.*
42. Ziegler JL, Deisseroth AB, Appelbaum FR, *et al*: Burkitt's lymphoma — a model for intensive chemotherapy. *Sem Oncol 4:317–323, 1977.*

CHAPTER NINE

Bone Marrow and CNS Involvement in Non-Hodgkin's Lymphoma

MICHAEL WILLOUGHBY, MD

INTRODUCTION: RELATIONSHIP OF NON-HODGKIN'S LYMPHOMA TO ACUTE LYMPHOID LEUKEMIA

THE OUTSTANDING CLINICAL feature of undifferentiated lymphoma, non-Burkitt's type, is the propensity for leukemic change.[1] In the particular series referred to by Sullivan,[1] the bone marrow eventually became involved in 21 out of 30 patients (70%) and in 10 out of the 11 presenting with mediastinal mass.[2] Ten out of the 21 children with bone marrow infiltration also developed CNS involvement. A much lower incidence of bone marrow and CNS infiltration occurred in patients with initial intestinal presentation in this and in other series.

If it is accepted as a working hypothesis that at least some of the subsets of childhood non-Hodgkin's lymphoma (NHL) are in fact *the same disease* as corresponding subsets of acute lymphoid leukemia (ALL), then the high incidence of bone marrow and CNS involvement is to be expected. Consistent with this hypothesis are the following three observations: (1) the association of mediastinal mass both with leukemic transformation in non-Hodgkin's lymphoma (Table 3) and with T-cell acute lymphoid leukemia[3]; (2) the tendency for non-Burkitt, undifferentiated malignant lymphoma to transform into acute lymphoid leukemia and the tendency for histiocytic lymphomas to transform to acute monocytic leukemia (Table 2); and (3) the presence of similar biological markers in non-Hodgkin's lymphoma and acute lymphoid leukemia, including terminal transferase in cells from lymphoblastic lymphomas[4] and in "common" and T-cell ALL[5,6] and the similarity of immunological membrane markers, whether T-cell, B-cell, or null-cell, in non-Hodgkin's lymphoma and in leukemia.[7-12] Kersey

Department of Paediatric Haematology/Oncology, Royal Hospital for Sick Children, Yorkhill, Glasgow G3 8SJ, and Faculty of Medicine, University of Glasgow, Glasgow, Scotland

TABLE 1
Biological Relationships Between Subsets of Non-Hodgkin's Lymphoma and Leukemia

Lymphoma phase	Membrane markers	Leukemic phase
Non-Burkitt, especially with mediastinal mass (Sternberg's sarcoma) (DLPD, DM, DU)	HTLA E + ve	T-cell ALL
Non-Burkitt, usually without mediastinal mass (DLPD, DM, DU)	Ia "Common" ALL	"Common" ALL
Burkitt (DU)	Ia, SIg	B-cell ALL
Diffuse histiocytic (DH)	Histiocytic markers	Acute monocytic leukemia

Abbreviations: DLPD, diffuse lymphocytic, poorly differentiated; DU, diffuse undifferentiated; DH, diffuse histiocytic; DM, diffuse mixed (lymphocytic and histiocytic); E + ve, sheep erythrocyte positive; SIg, surface immunoglobulin; HTLA, human thymus leukemia antigen.

et al.[13] have particularly emphasized the unity of childhood T-cell acute lymphoid leukemia and non-Hodgkin's lymphoma, both having a predominantly lymphatic or thymic extramedullary origin. They emphasize the separation of T-cell ALL from both common ALL of bone marrow origin and from B-cell leukemia and Burkitt's lymphoma, which is also predominantly extramedullary in origin.

We can now see (Table 1) that non-Burkitt's lymphoma in childhood includes subsets with the same membrane markers as T-cell leukemia or "common" ALL. The non-Burkitt's lymphomas having T-cell membrane markers also have the well-recognized associations of both mediastinal mass (Fig. 1) and a predilection to early CNS involvement. Similarly, acute monocytic leukemia represents the leukemic phase of diffuse histiocytic lymphoma, and B-cell ALL represents the leukemic phase of Burkitt-type lymphoma.

These interrelationships have emerged particularly clearly from the retrospective clinical and pathological study of children with non-Hodgkin's lymphoma by Pinkel *et al.*[14] (Table 2). As in most other studies of non-Hodgkin's lymphoma, a basic criterion for diagnosis was that the bone marrow must not be overtly involved. Subsequently, there was a high incidence of bone marrow involvement (32%) and CNS involvement (26%), either as the first focus of relapse or as a later progression of the disease. In some children bone marrow relapse preceded CNS involvement, in others the CNS relapse preceded bone marrow involvement, or leukemic transformation. Fifteen out of the 62 patients (24%) died with leukemia. There was a lower incidence of CNS and bone marrow involvement in stage I

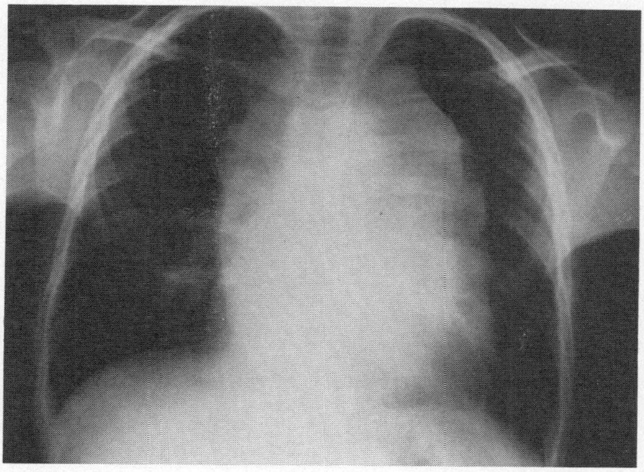

FIG. 1. Chest x-ray showing mediastinal mass at presentation in a boy of 12 with T-cell NHL. Eighteen months later he developed bilateral testicular infiltration, with later CNS and marrow involvement.

disease, and none in two additional patients with nodular lymphoma. Within the group of patients with diffuse non-Burkitt's lymphoma, 8 out of the 14 with marrow involvement eventually had CNS involvement. This rate of occurrence of CNS involvement is about the same as would be expected in children with ALL who were not given CNS prophylaxis. One child developed CNS, bone marrow, and testicular infiltration. Pinkel and his colleagues concluded from this study that what is called diffuse, undifferentiated, non-Burkitt's type lymphoma is actually acute lymphoid leukemia without apparent invasion of bone marrow and peripheral blood by neoplastic lymphocytes at the time of diagnosis. Similarly, diffuse, histiocytic lymphoma is acute monocytic leukemia without overt marrow or blood invasion. They point out that one could equally say that acute lymphoid leukemia and acute monocytic leukemia are stage IV lymphomas. This concept is central to current concepts regarding the pathogenesis of bone marrow and CNS involvement in childhood non-Hodgkin's lymphoma.

DEFINITION OF BONE MARROW AND CNS INVOLVEMENT

Current lack of uniformity in defining leukemia as opposed to stage IV non-Hodgkin's lymphoma makes interpretation of results of therapy extremely difficult.[21] In spite of the conceptual difficulties in separating non-Hodgkin's lymphoma from leukemia, it is nevertheless useful, actually vital for the purpose of staging, to determine whether the bone marrow is involved at diagnosis or not.

Wollner *et al.*[15] have proposed a simplified staging system for childhood non-Hodgkin's lymphoma in which the defining criteria for stage IV disease are bone marrow and/or CNS involvement. Because of possible "patchy" infiltration,

TABLE 2
Development of Bone Marrow and CNS Involvement in Non-Hodgkin's Lymphoma[a]

Diffuse malignant lymphoma: 62 children			
	Total number of patients	Total number BM or CNS involvement	Relapse or extension of disease
Undifferentiated, non-Burkitt (DLPD)			
Stage I	8	1	BM (1), extended to CNS, died of ALL
Stage II	18	8	BM (1), extended to CNS, died of ALL; CNS (4), extended to BM (2), late extension to BM (3), died of ALL (3)
Stage III	13	6	BM (1), died of ALL; CNS (5), extended to BM (4), died of ALL (3)
Stage IV	2	2	Extension to BM (2), died of ALL (2)
Subtotals	41	17 (41%)	
Undifferentiated, possible Burkitt's lymphoma			
Stages I and II	2	2	CNS (1); Extended to BM (1), died of ALL
Histiocytic (DH) lymphoma			
Stage I	3	0	
Stage II	7	4	BM (1), died of AMOL; CNS (3)
Stages III and IV	9	4	BM (3), died of AMOL; CNS (1), died of AMOL
Totals	62	27 (43%)	BM only (11); CNS only (7); BM and CNS (9)

[a]Data from Pinkel *et al.*, ref. 14.

Wollner and associates have made it their policy to aspirate bone marrow from at least three different sites. If the bone marrow smears are suspicious but not diagnostic, then a marrow biopsy is performed. It is believed that histologic sections of the bone marrow are superior to smears for detection of lymphoma.[16,17] Wollner *et al.*[15] found that about 10% of their cases showed clumps of lymphoma cells in only one or two of the three aspirates. Discordant results from different sites of marrow sampling have likewise occasionally been recorded even in ALL, where there is typically a much heavier and more uniform infiltration.[18] At Stanford, the policy since 1964 has been to perform marrow biopsy for histological examination by either Westerman-Jensen or Jamshidi techniques or by open bone marrow biopsy.[19] Ideally, one would like to use multiple sampling sites and have histology, cytology, cytochemistry, and membrane marker determinations of any positive infiltrate. Cytology can be obtained from trephine "touch" imprints[20] as well as from the more usual smears of aspirated bone marrow. If a specimen for study of membrane markers is to be obtained from involved bone marrow, this requires aspiration of the specimen directly into a heparinized tissue culture medium. There are, however, practical and ethical limitations to the number and types of bone marrow punctures that can be performed in young children without submitting the child to general anesthesia.

It is a question of semantics whether bone marrow infiltration at diagnosis signifies stage IV non-Hodgkin's lymphoma or alters the diagnosis to one of acute leukemia.[14] Recognizing this dilemma, Pinkel *et al.* regard absence of diffuse infiltration of the bone marrow or peripheral blood at the time of initial presentation as a prerequisite for the diagnosis of non-Hodgkin's lymphoma. Murphy has suggested that the presence of 25% tumor cells in the initial bone marrow differential is a convenient dividing line between non-Hodgkin's lymphoma and leukemia.[21] Carabell *et al.*[22] used a figure of 5% blast cells to make this distinction between NHL and leukemia. Presence of circulating blast cells in the peripheral blood, at the time when the patient is first seen, is easier to interpret and has been used to exclude the diagnosis of non-Hodgkin's lymphoma.[19] Wollner *et al.*[15] have used slightly different diagnostic criteria, however, since they included a small number of patients with circulating blast cells within their category of non-Hodgkin's lymphoma.

Bone marrow relapse or progression to later marrow involvement is easier to define by comparing the relapse bone marrow smears with the smears obtained at the time of diagnosis. Hutter *et al.*[23] regarded the presence of greater than 5% blasts as diagnostic of bone marrow relapse. On the other hand, Fitzpatrick *et al.*[24] used a figure of 25% blasts to define the presence of bone marrow relapse. Marrow relapse progresses to a leukemic blood picture in a significant proportion of patients, particularly those with diffuse lymphocytic, poorly differentiated lymphomas,[19] but not necessarily in patients with Burkitt's histology.[25] In most earlier studies, it was this *leukemic transformation* that was recorded. For practical purposes, leukemic transformation can be regarded as synonymous with the development of bone marrow involvement.

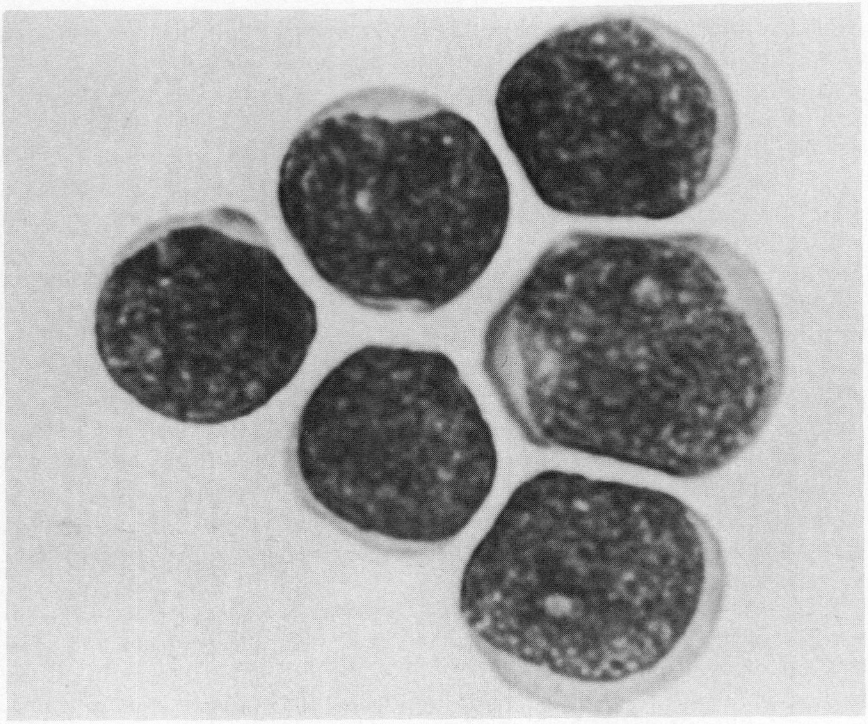

FIG. 2 Leukemic cells identified in the CSF of a child with NHL using the Cytospin method (Leishman stain, ×3000).

CNS involvement is clinically suspected from the development of symptoms and signs of increased intracranial pressure or cranial nerve paralysis as in a child with acute leukemia. CNS involvement is confirmed by pleocytosis of 10 or more nucleated cells/mm^3 in the absence of gross blood contamination or infection.[24] Watanabe *et al.*[2] found CSF cell counts between 31 and 17,900/mm^3 (median 1920/mm^3), elevated CSF protein (greater than 40 mg/dl) in five out of seven patients (range 25–988 mg/dl, median 74), and CSF glucose less than 35 mg/dl in three out of seven patients. These criteria are similar to those used to diagnose CNS involvement in acute leukemia.[26]

Watanabe *et al.*[2] and Bunn *et al.*[27] required (1) the presence of clinical symptoms suggestive of increased intracranial pressure together with (2) the presence in the CSF of cells with morphological features of abnormal or immature lymphoreticular cells, even if the number of cells in the CSF is not increased. Cytology can be assessed from stained films made by the Cytospin technique[28,29] or by another concentration method (Fig. 2). By this technique one can distinguish between lymphomatous infiltration and a viral meningitis, such as herpes zoster, to

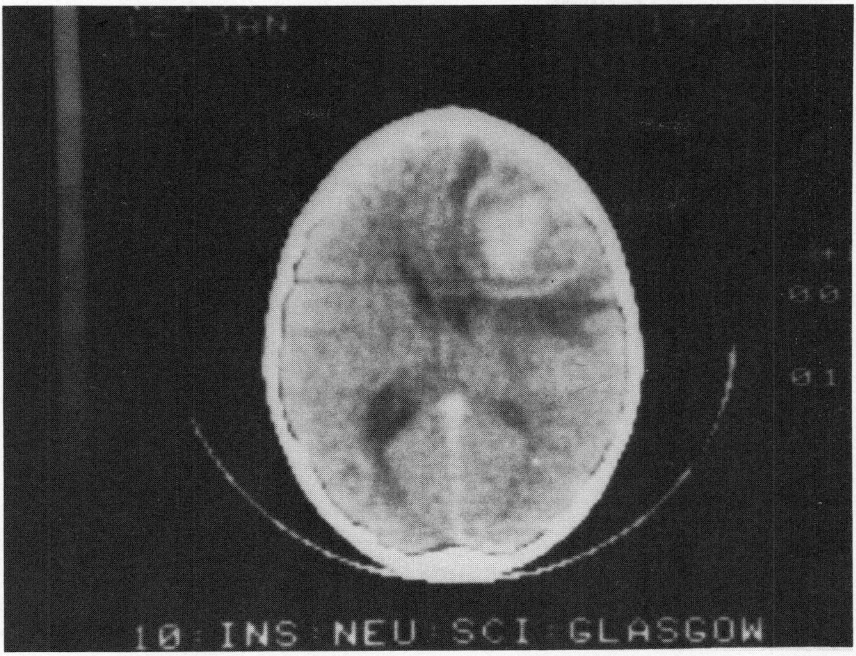

FIG. 3 CAT scan (EMI scan) showing probable intracranial hematoma in a 10-year-old girl with T-cell leukemia lymphoma and neurological syndrome but negative CSF cytology. She subsequently showed good neurological recovery.

which patients with lymphoma are prone. Also, one may detect lymphomatous or leukemic involvement of the CNS at an earlier stage, before a pleocytosis has developed. Even one malignant cell/mm^3 of CSF corresponds to 1000 cells/ml, which would represent a significant CNS infiltration. In certain instances, it is possible to augment the conventional Romanowsky stains (such as Wright's, Leishman, or May-Grunwald Giemsa stain) by cytochemical stains, such as PAS or acid phosphatase, which are of value in identifying T-cell lymphoblasts.[30] In a recent patient whose CSF showed pleocytosis (6900 blasts/mm^3), it was possible to collect sufficient cells for independent membrane marker studies. It was shown that virtually 100% of the cells formed rosettes with sheep erythrocytes. (These assays were kindly performed by Dr. Janossy in London.) This patient was a four-year-old boy who had presented eight months earlier with a mediastinal mass (Fig. 1) diagnosed as a Sternberg sarcoma; the peripheral blood count was normal, but bone marrow involvement was present.

More problematical are occasional patients who have neurological symptoms but whose CSF cytology is normal.[19] Further investigations including CT scans are indicated to exclude the possibility of deep brain involvement by lymphoma, hematoma, or abscess (Fig. 3). Although lymphomatous involvement of the brain

TABLE 3
Bone Marrow Involvement in Childhood Non-Hodgkin's Lymphoma Related to Primary Site of Disease

Primary site			References
Mediastinal	Intestinal	Peripheral lymph node	
10/11	1/8	5/5	Watanabe *et al.*[2]
2/3	1/10		Aghai *et al.*[33]
9/11	1/6		Glatstein *et al.*[19]
6/12	1/9	3/5	Hutter *et al.*[23]
8/22	2/7	2/14	Pinkel *et al.*[14]
7/16	1/18	2/20	Carabell *et al.*[22]
42/75 (56%)	7/58 (12%)	12/44 (27%)	

is probably rare in the absence of positive CSF cytology, this remains a possibility in non-Hodgkin's lymphoma, as indeed has recently been described in adults with acute myeloid leukemia.[31] In general, the CNS involvement that occurs in children with non-Hodgkin's lymphoma is primarily arachnoidal.[14] These CNS lesions may have a similar mode of evolution and spread as those seen in CNS involvement by ALL,[32] with deep brain involvement developing only at a late stage. Results of using regimens for prevention of CNS involvement have, however, been generally less satisfactory in non-Hodgkin's lymphoma than in acute lymphoid leukemia.[21,46]

INCIDENCE OF MARROW INVOLVEMENT: RELATION TO CLINICAL PRESENTATION, STAGING, AND HISTOLOGICAL TYPE

At diagnosis, Wollner *et al.*[15] included among their 86 children with non-Hodgkin's lymphoma 26 (30%) with marrow involvement. These 26 patients were classified as stage IV disease. In 12 patients there were <25% blasts, in 5 patients there were 25–50% of blasts, and 9 patients showed greater than 50% of blasts. The latter group was associated with variable degrees of anemia, thrombocytopenia, and circulating blast cells. Glatstein *et al.*[19] included 5 out of 31 with focal marrow involvement but no circulating blasts as being stage IV non-Hodgkin's lymphoma. Agha *et al.*[33] included 3 out of 17, and Hausner *et al.*[34] included 3 out of 30. Other series, such as that of Hutter *et al.*[23] included no instances of bone marrow involvement at diagnosis, while Pinkel *et al.*[14] and Carabell *et al.*[22] excluded such cases by definition.

Of equal clinical importance is the high frequency of later progression to bone marrow involvement and leukemic transformation in patients with apparently normal bone marrow at diagnosis. Jones and Klingbert[35] reviewed the early series

TABLE 4
Bone Marrow Involvement in Childhood Non-Hodgkin's Lymphoma Related to Cell Type or Histological Classification

Non-Burkitt type, includes DLPD, DM, DU, and T-cell convoluted	Burkitt's type, includes probable case	Histiocytic type, includes DH	References[a]
21/30	2/13	1/8	Watanabe *et al.*[2]
			Sullivan[1]
3/7[b]	0/8	0/2	Aghai *et al.*[33]
10/18[c]		3/13[d]	Glatstein *et al.*[19]
10/24		0/2	Hutter *et al.*[23]
14/41	1/2	3/19	Pinkel *et al.*[14]
5/26	1/2	0/3	Murphy *et al.*[36]
5/13	0/5	1/8	Landberg *et al.*[51]
5/16[d]	3/10+	0/4	Hausner *et al.*[34]
73/175 (42%)	7/40 (18%)	8/59 (14%)	Total 88/274 (32%)

Adult diffuse NHL (DLPD)	Adult histiocytic (DH)	References
27%	5%	Jones *et al.*[17]
29%	5%	Dick *et al.*[20]
30%	9%	Rosenberg[52]
61%	17%	Stein *et al.*[38]

[a]In these series there was a total of 7 patients with nodular histology, none of whom showed marrow involvement.
[b]All 3 present at diagnosis.
[c]Includes 4 present at diagnosis.
[d]Includes 1 present at diagnosis.

published between 1953 and 1962 which, together with their own patients, showed 62 of 208 (30%) developing leukemic transformation. More recent studies employing contemporary staging, follow-up, and longer survival are shown in Tables 3 and 4. The overall incidence of bone marrow involvement in childhood non-Hodgkin's lymphoma in these eight series is 32% (Table 4), which is very close to the figure of 30% derived from earlier series. Development of marrow relapse has been related to site of primary lymphoma (Table 3), histology of lymphoma (Table 4), and preceding intensive chemotherapy.

In early studies it was recognized that there was an unusually high incidence of bone marrow involvement in patients presenting with mediastinal mass and a lesser incidence of bone marrow involvement in those with intestinal presentation.[35] This pattern has been confirmed in recent series (Table 3). Combining six such reports, 56% of children with a mediastinal mass at presentation developed bone marrow involvement, compared to 27% in those presenting with cervical or other peripheral lymph node enlargement. Only 12% of children with primary intestinal lymphoma, usually ileum, caecum, or colon, developed bone marrow relapse. These differences cannot be explained solely by the fact that intestinal and peripheral nodal lymphoma are commonly more localized, since patients presenting with mediastinal mass also commonly have only stage I or stage II disease.[36] Five out of six patients with stage I or stage II non-Hodgkin's (non-Burkitt's) lymphoma with mediastinal masses developed leukemia in the M. D. Anderson series.[1] Four of 10 children with stage II disease and mediastinal mass developed bone marrow involvement, while three of six children with stage III disease and mediastinal mass developed bone marrow involvement in the series of Pinkel *et al.*[14] Nevertheless, it is true that a mediastinal mass is seldom associated with stage I disease, since it is usually accompanied by cervical or axillary lymph node enlargement or pleural spread; and stage I disease rarely involves the bone marrow. In the St. Jude study (Table 2), only one out of eight children with stage I non-Burkitt's lymphoma later developed marrow involvement, compared to half of those with stage II or stage III, and two out of two with stage IV disease developed bone marrow involvement.

Incidence of marrow involvement also varies according to histological type of non-Hodgkin's lymphoma (Table 4). In childhood, this is almost invariably *diffuse,* and in the rare instances of *nodular* histology, marrow involvement must be extremely rare. The commonest type of childhood non-Hodgkin's lymphoma is the non-Burkitt's lymphocytic lymphoma, which by Rappaport's classification includes diffuse lymphocytic and poorly differentiated, diffuse mixed (lymphocytic and histiocytic), and diffuse undifferentiated histologies, and by Lukes and Collins's (1974)[37] classification includes T-cell and convoluted cell types.[36] Burkitt's lymphoma and histiocytic lymphoma are less common. There is some cross correlation, since mediastinal presentation is seen predominantly among the non-Burkitt, T-cell type, but a small number of histiocytic cases can also present in this way.[1] Intestinal cases have a higher proportion of B-cell, including Burkitt-type lymphomas. The higher incidence of bone marrow involvement in non-Burkitt type (42%) compared to Burkitt's (18%) and histiocytic (14%) is compatible with the common sites of presentation of these histological types.

Adult and childhood non-Hodgkin's lymphomas show a rather similar overall incidence of marrow involvement within the histological categories of diffuse lymphocytic and histiocytic lymphomas (Table 4). Nevertheless, the pattern of the adult disease is entirely different in two respects. First, this involvement occurs predominantly at diagnosis. Among 121 adult patients, infiltration was present initially in 44 and developed later in only 5.[38] Second, patients with nodular histology show a similar[38] or higher[39] incidence of bone marrow involvement compared to those with diffuse histology. Also, the relatively rare well-differentiated diffuse lymphocytic lymphoma, unknown in childhood, showed initial involvement in all of seven patients (100%) in these two adult series. Actual leukemia, as opposed to marrow involvement, may be much lower in adults

TABLE 5
•Incidence of CNS Involvement in Childhood Non-Hodgkin's Lymphoma Related to Marrow Involvement, Including Comparison with Adults

	Marrow involvement present	Marrow involvement absent	References
Children	10/21[a]	0/9	Watanabe *et al.*[2]
	1/3	3/14	Aghai *et al.*[33]
	14/26[b]	3/15	Fitzpatrick *et al.*[24]
	4/10[c]	2/16	Hutter *et al.*[23]
	12/32[d]	7/32	Pinkel *et al.*[14]
	4/6[c]	6/25	Murphy *et al.*[36]
	16/6	2/21	Landberg *et al.*[50]
	6/9	3/21	Hausner *et al.*[34]
	52/113 (46%)	26/153 (17%)	Total 78/266 (29%)
Adults	19/47 (40%)	3/43 (7%)	Gendelman *et al.* [41]
			Total 22/90 (24%)

[a]2 Prior to bone marrow involvement.
[b]1 Prior to bone marrow involvement.
[c]3 Prior to bone marrow involvement.
[d]7 Prior to bone marrow involvement.

compared to children. In 1200 adults, Rosenberg *et al.*[40] found 88 instances of leukemic transformation, of which five were acute leukemia, 34 chronic lymphocytic leukemia, and 49 "leukolymphosarcoma."

CNS INVOLVEMENT: RELATION TO MARROW INFILTRATION, CLINICAL PRESENTATION, STAGING, AND HISTOLOGICAL TYPE

The high incidence of meningeal involvement in childhood non-Hodgkin's lymphoma, with clinical and CSF findings similar to meningeal leukemia, was clearly documented by Watanabe *et al.*[2] and has been confirmed in subsequent pediatric series (Table 5). The overall incidence of meningeal involvement in childhood non-Hodgkin's lymphoma is close to 30%. In the Houston study, CNS involvement was confined to those showing bone marrow infiltration; CNS involvement preceded the bone marrow infiltration in three patients and followed the bone marrow infiltration in seven patients. In the other series, this association is still apparent, but bone marrow infiltration has not been a necessary prerequisite for CNS involvement. Again the CNS disease preceded bone marrow infiltration in a minority. This possibility was emphasized by Hutter *et al.*,[23] who found CNS involvement before or without bone marrow infiltration in five out of six instances. This argues against the previously held view that circulation of blast cells in the

TABLE 6
CNS Involvement in Childhood Non-Hodgkin's Lymphoma Related to Site of Primary Disease

Mediastinal		Intestinal	References
Present	Absent	Present	
5/11	5/19	0/8	Watanabe *et al.*[2]
1/3	3/14	3/10[a]	Aghai *et al.*[33]
2/11	1/20	1/6	Glatstein *et al.*[19]
6/12	0/14	0/9	Hutter *et al.*[23]
8/21	11/43	3/16	Pinkel *et al.*[14]
1/5	9/28		Murphy *et al.*[36]
3/10	6/20	3/8[a]	Hausner *et al.*[34]
26/73 (36%)	35/156 (22%)	10/57 (18%)	

[a]All three had Burkitt's lymphoma.

blood was the route by which CNS involvement occurred. By comparison, adult non-Hodgkin's lymphoma shows a slightly lower incidence of CNS disease (24%), but again with a higher incidence in those with marrow involvement.[41]

Since there are associations between CNS and bone marrow disease (Table 5), and between bone marrow and mediastinal disease (Table 3), it is not surprising that CNS involvement develops more frequently in those presenting with a mediastinal mass. This relationship was first noted by Watanabe *et al.*[2] and a similar trend is found by pooling results of other recent series (Table 6). By contrast, no instances of CNS involvement were found among 17 children presenting with intestinal lymphoma,[2,23] none of whom had received CNS prophylaxis. Other series have shown a small number of intestinal cases with CNS involvement (Table 6), six of the nine having Burkitt's lymphoma. Apart from Burkitt's lymphoma patients, there is a remarkably low incidence of CNS involvement from intestinal non-Hodgkin's lymphoma, particularly in stage I or stage II disease, or if the tumor is totally resectable.[42]

By relating CNS involvement to histology or cell type, one finds a high incidence (42%) in Burkitt's lymphoma, not only in the series of Nkruma and Perkins,[43] but also in other series (Table 7). Ziegler *et al.*[44] similarly reported a 46% incidence of CNS involvement in Burkitt's lymphoma. One-third of children with non-Burkitt's lymphoma developed CNS disease, while this is infrequent (9%) in histiocytic lymphoma in children. This contrasts with the situation in adults, where there appears to be a predilection for CNS involvement in diffuse histiocytic lymphoma.[45] Gendelman *et al.*[41] reported a 60% incidence of CNS involvement in adults with this lymphoma (reticulum cell sarcoma), while Bunn *et al.*[27] reported a 29% incidence in adults with diffuse histiocytic lymphoma.

Stage of disease at diagnosis is also related to incidence of CNS involvement and bone marrow infiltration in both the non-Burkitt's and diffuse histiocytic types of

TABLE 7
CNS Involvement in Childhood Non-Hodgkin's Lymphoma Related to Histological or Cell Types

Non-Burkitt type, includes DLPD, DM, DU, and T-cell convoluted	Burkitt's type, includes probable cases	Histiocytic type, includes DH	References
10/30			Watanabe *et al.*[2]
3/7	3/8	0/2	Aghai *et al.*[33]
2/19		1/13	Glatstein *et al.*[19]
11/19		2/24	Fitzpatrick *et al.*[24]
5/20		0/2	Hutter *et al.*[23]
16/41	1/2	2/19	Pinkel *et al.*[14]
5/16	4/10	0/4	Hausner *et al.*[34]
	19/45		Nkrumah and Perkins[43]
52/152 (34%)	27/65 (42%)	5/54 (9%)	

childhood non-Hodgkin's lymphoma (Table 2). In a series of children at St. Jude Children's Research Hospital with localized favorable stage I disease at presentation, there was a less than 10% risk of developing the first relapse in the CNS.[21] In a similar series in Boston, none out of 15 patients showed occurrence of first relapse in the CNS.[22] Identification of these categories of non-Hodgkin's lymphoma in which there is a low incidence of CNS disease is as important as identifying the high-risk mediastinal, T-cell and Burkitt's cases, when considering the justification for CNS prophylaxis in different subgroups of the disease.

PATHOGENESIS AND POSSIBLE PROPHYLACTIC THERAPY

Bone marrow and CNS relapse in childhood non-Hodgkin's lymphoma constitute major obstacles to the long-term control and cure of the disease.[21,22] Recurrence at the site of original primary tumor is rare after adequate local radiotherapy.[14] Possible approaches to the prevention of bone marrow and CNS relapse, and thus an improved survival rate, depend upon our concepts regarding their pathogenesis. Is there some degree of marrow involvement at diagnosis in all children with non-Hodgkin's lymphoma, bearing in mind the close connection with acute leukemia? Is the CNS seeded (1) at presentation, (2) at the time of bone marrow or blood invasion, or (3) as part of late extension of progressive uncontrolled disease?

The answer to the first question is that the bone marrow is uninvolved in at least 50% of cases of apparent stage I disease, since about 50% long-term survival is obtained after local radiotherapy alone.[19] In stage II and stage III disease (using the Ann Arbor classification), the lower survival rate after local therapy suggests correspondingly lower proportions of patients with uninvolved bone marrow (30–40%). In stage IV or disseminated disease, the marrow is involved in almost all cases,[15] and long-term survival is virtually nil with conventional therapy.[19] The LSA2-L2 protocol is an intensive multidrug chemotherapy program similar to but more aggressive than the chemotherapy regimen of proven efficacy in childhood ALL. When the LSA2-L2 protocol was given in combination with appropriate radiotherapy to sites of bulky disease, there was reduced incidence of marrow relapse to 1 out of 43 (2.5%) compared to 25 out of 43 (58.5%) seen in conventionally treated control patients.[15] Survival rate increased from 11 to 76% at a median observation time of over 25 months.

Pathogenesis of CNS involvement

Seeding at presentation is unlikely to be the sole mechanism in view of the relative failure of prophylaxis with cranial irradiation plus intrathecal methotrexate. Thus 5 out of 23 such patients with mediastinal tumors and leukemia developed CNS disease as their initial relapse on therapy[21]; three of seven patients with non-Burkitt's lymphoma given CNS prophylaxis developed CNS involvement, compared to three out of four not given CNS prophylaxis.[46]

Seeding at the time of bone marrow or blood involvement was supported by the early impression that CNS involvement was confined to patients with marrow infiltration.[2] But the observations of Hutter *et al.*[23] and of others (Table 5) showed that the CNS can be involved without accompanying bone marrow infiltration.

It is possible that this form of extramedullary relapse represents spread due to failure to achieve systemic control of the tumor; this mechanism is also suggested as a possible explanation for testicular relapse in ALL.[47] This concept is supported by the lower incidence of CNS relapse in patients given intensive systemic chemotherapy. Wollner *et al.*[15] reported a lower rate of CNS involvement, 7 out of 43 (16%), in patients treated with the LSA2-L2 protocol, compared to 15 out of 43 (35%) in a nonprotocol group, some of whom had received CNS irradiation, but without subsequent combination chemotherapy. The LSA2-L2 protocol included repeated courses of intrathecal methotrexate. Using both early CNS prophylaxis and also intensive chemotherapy, Weinstein *et al.*[48] have apparently eliminated CNS involvement in 31 consecutive children with non-Hodgkin's lymphoma by combination of early multidrug chemotherapy (vincristine, prednisolone, adriamycin, and L-asparaginase) followed by cranial irradiation plus intrathecal methotrexate and subsequent multidrug pulse maintenance. In their historical controls, treated similarly, but without CNS prophylaxis or the adriamycin combination chemotherapy, 9 out of 36 (25%) developed CNS disease.[22]

Burkitt's lymphoma, however, may involve the CNS by a different route than other forms of childhood non-Hodgkin's lymphoma. Direct extension from involved adjacent sites, i.e., facial bones, extradural sites, peripheral and cranial nerves, has been proposed on the basis of autopsy findings.[44] This may explain the failure of intrathecal methotrexate[49] or craniospinal irradiation[50] to prevent CNS relapse in this specific form of non-Hodgkin's lymphoma.

In conclusion, it would appear that the most hopeful current approach to prevention of bone marrow and CNS relapse in non-Hodgkin's lymphoma is the use of intensive systemic chemotherapy from the outset, perhaps with early additional chemotherapy or radiotherapy directed to the CNS in patients in high-risk categories. CNS prophylaxis alone is of limited and unproven value.

SUMMARY

Childhood non-Hodgkin's lymphoma and acute leukemia are closely related. The overall incidence of bone marrow involvement in non-Hodgkin's lymphoma is approximately 30%. The incidence of bone marrow involvement is higher (56%) in patients presenting with mediastinal mass, and lower (12%) in those with intestinal lymphoma. The incidence of bone marrow involvement is higher in patients with non-Burkitt's malignant lymphoma (42%) than in those with Burkitt's lymphoma (18%) or histiocytic lymphoma (14%).

CNS involvement also develops in close to 30% of patients. CNS involvement is strongly, but not exclusively, associated with preceding bone marrow infiltration and also with the finding of a mediastinal mass at presentation. There is a particularly high incidence of CNS involvement (42%) in Burkitt's lymphoma. Both bone marrow and CNS involvement constitute major obstacles to cure. Conventional CNS prophylaxis is of limited value. However, intensification of systemic chemotherapy appears to reduce the incidence of both bone marrow and CNS relapse, with resulting improved survival.

References

1. Sullivan, MP: Non-Hodgkin's lymphoma of childhood, in Sutow WW, Vietti TJ, Fernbach DJ (ed.): *Clinical Pediatric Oncology*. C. V. Mosby, St. Louis, 1973, pp. 313–334.
2. Watanabe A, Sullivan MP, Sutow WW, Wilbur JH: Undifferentiated lymphoma, non-Burkitt's type; meningeal and bone marrow involvement in children. *Am J Dis Child 125:57–61, 1973*.
3. Sen L, Borella L: Clinical importance of lymphoblasts with T markers in childhood leukemia. *N Engl J Med 292:828–832, 1975*.
4. Donlon JA, Jaffe ES, Braylan RC: Terminal deoxynucleotidyl transferase activity in malignant lymphomas. *N Engl J Med 297:461–464, 1977*.
5. McCaffrey R, Harrison TA, Parkman R, Baltimore D: Terminal deoxynucleotidyl transferase activity in human leukemic cells and in normal human thymocytes. *N Engl J Med 292:775–780, 1975*.
6. Hoffbrand AV, Ganeshaguru K, Janossy G, *et al*: Diagnostic value of TdT in acute leukemias. *Lancet 2:520–523, 1977*.
7. Kaplan J, Mastrangelo R, Peterson WD: Childhood lymphoblastic lymphoma, a cancer of thymus-derived lymphocytes. *Cancer Res 34:521–525, 1974*.
8. Gajl-Peczalska KJ, Bloomfield CD, Coccia PF: B- and T-cell lymphomas; analysis of blood and lymph nodes in 87 patients. *Am J Med 59:674–685, 1975*.

9. Flandrin G, Brouet JC, Daniel MT, Preud'homme JL: Acute leukemia with Burkitt's tumour cells; a study of six cases with special reference to lymphocyte markers. *Blood 45:183–188, 1975.*
10. Coccia PF, Kersey JH, Gajl-Peczalska KJ, *et al*: Prognostic significance of surface marker analysis in childhood non-Hodgkin's lymphoproliferative malignancies. *Am J Hematol 1:405–417, 1976.*
11. Jaffe ES, Braylan RC, Frank MM, *et al*: Heterogeneity of immunologic markers and surface morphology in childhood lymphoblastic lymphoma. *Blood 48:213–222, 1976.*
12. Seligmann M, Brouet JC, Preud'homme JL: Immunologic classification of non-Hodgkin's lymphomas; current status. *Cancer Treat Rep. 61:1179–1183, 1977.*
13. Kersey JH, Gajl-Peczalska KJ, Coccia PF, Nesbit ME: The nature of childhood leukemia and lymphoma. *Am J Pathol 90:487–495, 1978.*
14. Pinkel D, Johnson W, Aur RJA: Non-Hodgkin's lymphoma in children. *Br J Cancer 31:298–323, 1975.*
15. Wollner N, Burchenal JH, Lieberman PH, *et al*: Non-Hodgkin's lymphoma in children; a comparative study of two modalities of therapy. *Cancer 37:123–134, 1976.*
16. Liao KT: The superiority of histologic sections of aspirated bone marrow in malignant lymphomas; a review of 1124 examinations. *Cancer 27:618–628, 1971.*
17. Jones SE, Rosenberg SA, Kaplan HS: Non-Hodgkin's lymphomas. I Bone marrow involvement. *Cancer 29:954–960, 1972.*
18. Hann IM, Morris Jones PH, Evans DIK: Discrepancy of bone marrow aspirations in acute lymphoblastic leukemia in relapse. *Lancet 1:1215–1216, 1977.*
19. Glatstein E, Kim H, Donaldson SS, *et al*: Non-Hodgkin's lymphomas. VI. Results of treatment in childhood. *Cancer 34:204–211, 1974.*
20. Dick F, Bloomfield CD, Brunning RD: Incidence cytology and histopathology of non-Hodgkin's lymphomas in the bone marrow. *Cancer 33:1382–1398, 1974.*
21. Murphy SB: Prognostic features and obstacles for cure of childhood non-Hodgkin's lymphoma. *Sem Oncol 4:265–271, 1977.*
22. Carabell SC, Cassady JR, Weinstein HJ, Jaffe N: The role of radiation therapy in the treatment of pediatric non-Hodgkin's lymphomas. *Cancer 42:2193–2205, 1978.*
23. Hutter, JJ, Savara DE, Nelson M, Holn CP: Non-Hodgkin's lymphoma in children; correlation of CNS disease with initial presentation. *Cancer 36:2132–2137, 1975.*
24. Fitzpatrick J, Lieberman N, Sinks LF: Staging of acute leukemia and the relationship to CNS involvement; staging of ALL and CNS disease. *Cancer 33:1376–1381, 1974.*
25. Brunning RD, McKenna RW, Bloomfield CD, *et al*: Bone marrow involvement in Burkitt's lymphoma. *Cancer 40:1771–1779, 1977.*
26. Sullivan, MP, Vietti TJ, Fernbach DJ, *et al*: Clinical investigations in the treatment of meningeal leukemia; radiation therapy regimens vs. conventional intrathecal methotrexate. *Blood 34:301–319, 1969.*
27. Bunn PA Jr, Schein PS, Banks PM, De Vita VT Jr: Central nervous system complications in patients with diffuse histiocytic and undifferentiated lymphoma; leukemia revisited. *Blood 47:3–10, 1976.*
28. Komp DM: Cytocentrifugation in the management of central nervous system leukemia. *J Pediatr 81:992–994, 1972.*
29. Evans DIK, O'Rourke C, Morris Jones P: The cerebrospinal fluid in acute leukaemia of childhood; studies with the cytocentrifuge. *J Clin Pathol 27:226–230, 1974.*
30. Catovsky D: T-cell origin of acid-phosphatase-positive lymphoblasts. *Lancet 2:327–328, 1975.*
31. Pippard MJ, Callendar ST, Sheldon PWE: Infiltration of central nervous system in adult acute myeloid leukaemia. *Br Med J 1:227–279, 1979.*
32. Graham-Pole JR, Willoughby MLN: Leukemia in the nervous system; factors in pathogenesis. in Pochedly C, (ed): *Acute Childhood leukemia.* Modern Problems in Pediatrics series, Vol. 16. S. Karger, Basel, 1975, pp. 59–79.

33. Aghai Ee, Hulu N, Virag I, *et al*: Childhood non-Hodgkin's lymphoma; a study of 17 cases in Israel. *Cancer 33:1411–1418, 1974.*
34. Hausner RJ, Rosas-Uribe A, Wickstrum DA, Smith PC: Non-Hodgkin's lymphoma in the first two decades of life; a pathological study of 30 cases. *Cancer 40:1533–1547, 1977.*
35. Jones B, Klingbert WG: Lymphosarcoma in children; a report of 43 cases and review of the recent literature. *J Paediatr 63:11–20, 1963.*
36. Murphy SB, Frizzera G, Evans A: A study of childhood non-Hodgkin's lymphoma. *Cancer 36:2121–2131, 1975.*
37. Lukes RJ, Collins RD: Immunologic characterization of human malignant lymphomas. *Cancer 34:1488–1503, 1974.*
38. Stein RS, Ultmann JE, Byrne GE, *et al*: Bone marrow involvement in non-Hodgkin's lymphoma; implications for staging and therapy. *Cancer 37:629–636, 1976.*
39. Dick F, Bloomfield CD, Brunning RD: Incidence, cytology, and histopathology of non-Hodgkin's lymphomas in the bone marrow. *Cancer 33:1382–1398, 1974.*
40. Rosenberg SA, Diamond HD, Jaslowitz B, Craver LF: Lymphosarcoma; a review of 1269 cases. *Medicine* (Baltimore) *40:31–84, 1961.*
41. Gendelman S, Rizzo F, Mones RJ: Central nervous system complications of the leukemic conversion of the lymphomas. *Cancer 24:676–682, 1969.*
42. Nelson DR, Cassady JR, Traggis D, *et al*: The role of radiation therapy in localized resectable intestinal non-Hodgkin's lymphoma in children. *Cancer 39:89–97, 1977.*
43. Nkrumah FK, Perkins IV: Relapse in Burkitt's lymphoma. *Br J Cancer 17:455–460, 1976.*
44. Ziegler JL, Bluming AZ, Morrow RH, *et al*: Central nervous system involvement in Burkitt's lymphoma. *Blood 36:718–728, 1970.*
45. Bunn, PA Jr, Schein PS: Meningeal involvement in lymphoma. *N Engl J Med 290:517, 1974.*
46. Sullivan MP: Treatment of lymphoma. *Cancer 35:991–995, 1975.*
47. Baumer H, Mott MG, Gentle TA: Sex and prognosis in childhood acute lymphoblastic leukaemia. *Lancet 2:673–674, 1978.*
48. Weinstein H, Buell D, Cassady JR, *et al*: Improved prognosis for childhood non-Hodgkin's lymphoma (NHL). *Blood 50(suppl I):212, 1977.*
49. Ziegler JL, Bluming AZ: Intrathecal chemotherapy in Burkitt's lymphoma. *BR Med J 3:508–512, 1971.*
50. Olweny CLM, Atine I, Kaddu-Mukasa A: Prevention of meningeal relapse in Burkitt's lymphoma using craniospinal irradiation. *Semin Oncol 4:317–323, 1977.*
51. Landberg T, Garwicz S, Akerman M: Clinico-pathological study of non-Hodgkin's lymphomata in childhood. *Br J Cancer 31(suppl II):332–336, 1975.*
52. Rosenberg SA: Bone marrow involvement in the non-Hodgkin's lymphomata. *Br J Cancer 31(suppl II):261–264, 1975.*

CHAPTER TEN

Non-Hodgkin's Lymphomas in Children: An Overview

MARGARET P. SULLIVAN, MD

RECENT DISCOVERIES IN cellular immunology have provided insight into the fundamental nature of malignant lymphoid diseases, and real clues now exist as to possible modes of tumor induction. We are now able to readily identify cells of the T and B lymphatic systems, and we have an improved understanding of lymphocyte function in the two systems. These advances have influenced pathologic classification of the non-Hodgkin's lymphomas in a major way.[1,2] It is surprising that the new immunologic information has not yet significantly influenced therapy. LSA2-L2 regimen, an empirical treatment regimen has, however, markedly improved the prognosis of children with non-Hodgkin's lymphoma.[3,4] The combined and concurrent advances in immunology, classification, and treatment give promise of ultimate control, or eradication, of the lymphomatous diseases of childhood.

A major discovery in cellular immunology is the finding of rodent immune response genes located in the major histocompatibility complex. This immunological entity continues to be a matter of intense investigative study with promise of future clinical application.[5] Immune response genes have not yet been mapped in humans nor have specific gene products been identified as they have been in rodent systems. The B-cell neoplasm of African children, Burkitt's lymphoma, provides suggestive evidence that a genetic abberation in children with prior EB virus exposure may result in tumor induction. Stimuli that might act in concert with genetic perturbations so as to produce the same, or other lymphomas, in North American children have not been identified.

M.D. Anderson Hospital and Tumor Institute, and The University of Texas Cancer System, 6723 Bertner Drive, Houston, TX 77030

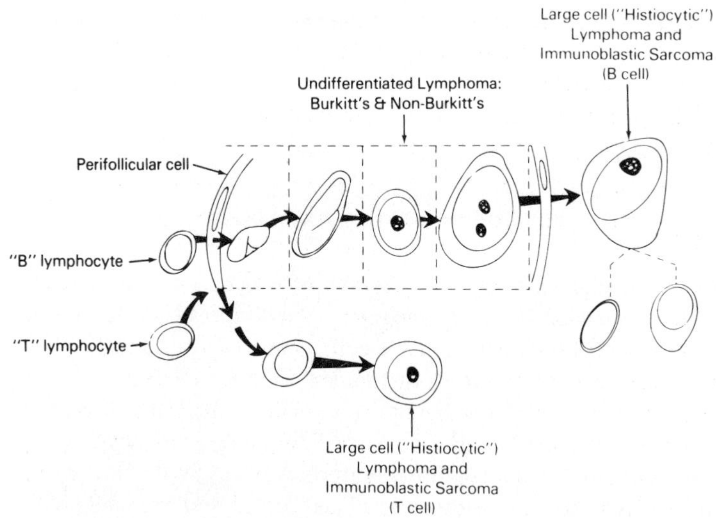

FIG. 1. Correlation of the transformation process with cytologic types of non-Hodgkin's lymphoma showing benign counterparts. The undifferentiated lymphomas, Burkitt's and non-Burkitt's types, represent tumors of the small, noncleaved follicular center cells (FCC) which occur in interfollicular tissues of lymph nodes. The large cell ("histiocytic") lymphoma and immunoblastic sarcoma (B-cell type) arise from B-immunoblasts in interfollicular tissue. The large ("histiocytic") lymphoma and immunoblastic sarcoma (Tcell type) arise from T immunoblasts in the interfollicular tissue. There is no benign counterpart of the lymphoblastic (convoluted) cell lymphoma in lymph nodes.

when applied to the non-Hodgkin's lymphomas of childhood that several alternate systems have been devised (see tabulation by Toledano and Meadows).[7] As noted by Ziegler,[8] staging proposals for Burkitt's lymphoma have been subjected to a series of revisions.

Many studies have also been devoted to characterizing "pure" leukemia, leukemia with large masses, lymphoma with bone marrow involvement, and "pure" lymphoma. Criteria have also been established to reflect the degree of bone marrow abnormality at diagnosis. These efforts to distinguish leukemia from lymphoma continue despite the fact that the degree of marrow involvement at diagnosis in T-cell lymphoma does not appear to affect either duration of remission or survival. The LSA2-L2 regimen is currently reported as producing over 80% disease-free survival across the spectrum of non-Hodgkin's lymphomas regardless of histologic and surface marker types. Survival has been similar in children whether they had less or more than 25% blasts in the bone marrow at diagnosis. As when using other treatment regimens, the clinical factors that most markedly limit the success of LSA2-L2 therapy appear to be (1) the extent and resectability of abdominal disease at diagnosis and (2) direct extensions of disease that invade the cranial vault and its contents. The importance of meticulous staging is also challenged by the often favorable course of convoluted cell disease involving the bone marrow and meninges at diagnosis. Likewise, at the other extreme, the value of staging is refuted by the frequency of disease extensions following treatment of localized lymphomas of all histologic types. A harder look at immunologic and functional attributes of lymphoid cells is indicated in order to achieve an understanding that will translate into more rational, specific therapy.

PATHOPHYSIOLOGY OF LYMPHOMAS

The older view that malignant cells exert their ill effects by "crowding out" normal cells must be abandoned, since malignant lymphoid cells are known to maintain the same mobility as normal lymphoid cells. Preservation of function has been documented, and in some instances maturation has been evident.

Lymphocytes are present in the blood in relatively small numbers; they leave the blood circuit freely to enter the lymphatic system.[10] In lambs, this physiologic circulation between blood and lymph develops during fetal life. Each immunologic type of lymphocyte has established and orderly traffic routes, with recirculation and population of en route tissues and organs. Lodging sites and traffic tempo differ for T cells and B cells.

T-cell characteristics

T cells are the more active; 70% are circulating and make four to six circuits daily.[1] Recognized lodging sites include the paracortical areas of lymph nodes, perivascular regions of the spleen, small foci in the gastrointestinal tract,[1] and the skin.[10] No information is available on the propensity for lodging in meninges or testicles, which are sites of obvious clinical interest that beg for investigation. A malignant clone might arise from a cell in transit or from a cell in any lodging site. The frequency of lymphoid tumor in a particular site should therefore relate to the number of cells homing to that site. Spread of T-cell diseases would therefore not be limited to extensions to contiguous nodes. In fact, T-cell disease extensions by way of blood-lymph circulation, recirculation, and homing would seem to be far more likely.

B-cell characteristics

Fewer B cells circulate. The tempo is slower since B cells are delayed in major capillary networks. Scattered cells are found in the bone marrow; the bulk of B cells reside in follicular centers of lymph nodes, the spleen, and the lamina propria of the gastrointestinal tract.[1,10] The major traffic is very specific. Thus immunoblasts from mesenteric lymph nodes preferentially home to abdominal nodes, which is in contrast to somatic immunoblasts, which home to spleen, lungs, and peripheral somatic lymph nodes.[11]

Homing of lymphoid cells

Homing, or *ecotaxis*, of lymphoid cells should be of particular interest to the oncologist. Cells of the lymphomyeloid system have the capacity to migrate preferentially and to arrange themselves in clear-cut microenvironments of peripheral lymphoid organs and tissues.[10] Many factors are known to influence homing; the most obvious would appear to be the home environment or stroma. Even the reticulin framework of the home appears to be of importance. The framework of the thymus differs from that of nodes in its openness. In addition, less reticulin is present in B-cell homing sites of lymph nodes, the spleen, and Peyer's patches.

A cell's ability to home can be altered by specific effector substances acting upon the cell surface membrane.[10] A partial list of these effector substances includes: neuraminidase, viral antigens, trypsin, conconavalin A, glycoproteins, lipopolysaccharides, a factor from the supernatant fluid from *Bordetella pertussis* cultures, and antilymphocyte antiserum. Exposure to these substances results in transient accumulations of lymphocytes in the liver, spleen, and pulmonary capillaries; entry into lymph nodes is reduced.

Alterations in the home also affect ecotaxis.[10] When an antigen is given intravenously, lymphoid cells are held up in the spleen. Whole body irradiation and stress act similarly. Antigen injected into a peripheral lymph node causes holdup in the first echelon nodes. When the home is altered locally or systemically, redistribution of lymphocytes between the lymphatic and vascular systems results.

The resident cells of a homing site participate in the homing attraction.[10] Homing sites contain two distinct types of dendritic cells which initiate the functional activities of lymphoid cells. Lymphocytes of different functional types are present. Among themselves the lymphocytes establish T-T and T-B interactions, which constitute a communications network with powerful immunoregulatory influences. Through these interactions, the type and intensity of an immune response is determined and autoimmune reactions are prevented.

ROLE OF T-CELL SUBPOPULATIONS

T-cell sets or subpopulations are important functionally in determining immune response.[12,13] In mice, T-cell subpopulations are identified by cell surface components (glycoprotein pattern) found on the cells during thymus-dependent differentiation. These surface components are not found on other tissues such as brain, kidney, liver, or spleen. They are specified by genes that are expressed exclusively during T-cell differentiation. These T-cell subpopulations have genetically assigned physiologic functions. In rodents the location of the genes controlling cell function has been determined. Although terminologies differ, the following "sets" are usually recognized: (1) helper or potentiator cells, (2) suppressor cells, (3) cytotoxic cells, and (4) regulatory cells.

Helper cells are described as sentinals, constantly screening other cells for antigens. Two populations exist.[16] The first assists B cells in producing antibodies and activates monocyte-macrophages for participation in delayed hypersensitivity responses. The antibody response is thus wholly dependent on active helper T cells, which regulate the quantity and quality of the antibody response. The second helper population activates B-cell immunoglobulin receptors by direct interaction with B cells. Each type of helper cell requires pro-helper cell action to initiate activity.

Suppressor cells also require a pro-suppressor cell for activation. Functionally these cells inhibit B-cell production of antibodies, suppress host resistance to tumors, suppress cytotoxic action, and terminate excessive responses, thus guarding against autoimmune reactions. Inhibition of antibody production by suppressor T cells has been demonstrated in a child with acute lymphocytic leukemia.[15] Marked decrease of levels of one or more of the immunoglobulins was present at diagnosis in several of our patients with convoluted cell lymphoma; this finding may be more common than had been previously expected in childhood non-Hodgkin's lymphomas. Cytotoxic cells destroy cells immunized to certain antigens as well as tumor cells. The regulatory cells, which constitute a pool that provides pro-helper cells and pro-suppressor cells, also regulate the supply and function of the more mature helper and suppressor cells.

All of the described characteristics that are manifested by abnormal lymphocytes must be accommodated if a staging system for non-Hodgkin's lymphoma in children is to be realistic and usable. The classical staging system for adult lymphomas, which spread by direct nodal extension or by a chance hematologic shower, has little applicability to lymphomas in children. Lymphomas in children are composed of rapidly dividing cells that may retain much of their natural mobility, variable functional capacity, and the ability to continue the maturation process. An even greater challenge is the identification and classification of those tumors in which the demonstrable abnormalities are secondary to a malignant T cell clone, which exerts its influence via the immunoregulatory network.[12-14]

FUTURE PROSPECTS IN THERAPY

The evolution of therapy for the non-Hodgkin's lymphomas of children and its current status have been described elsewhere in this volume by Mott.[17] Treatment has been, and still is, empirical. Past reliance on radiotherapy is now being augmented or replaced by an increasing emphasis on chemotherapy, in which cyclophosphamide plays a prominent role. In discussing immunologic strategies for the therapy of human neoplasia, Broder and Waldmann[14] emphasized the capacity of ionizing radiation to eliminate immunoregulatory cells and suppressor T cells. A similar result may follow debulking surgical procedures. Cyclophosphamide has also been shown to be effective in eliminating suppressor cell activity in a number of experimental situations.

An immunologic basis has been demonstrated for the therapeutic effectiveness of both 6-mercaptopurine and the adrenocortical steroids. Pretreatment with the purine analog (6-mercaptopurine) augments the humoral response to antigen, while the steroid analogs can eliminate precursors of suppressor cells. Other therapeutic suggestions include the use of peptidoglycan to increase the generation of carrier-specific helper cells, inactivation of suppressor cells by colchicine, and the use of indomethacin to counteract the excessive production of inhibitory prostaglandins by suppressor cells. The most intriguing suggestion[12-14] is the use of heteroantisera to eliminate undesirable suppressor T cells. This possibility will remain a theoretical consideration until such time as human suppressor cells and their factors are shown to express antigens encoded by a region analogous to the I-J chromosomal region of the major histocompatibility complex (H-2) in mice.

This decade has produced much new information for pediatric chemotherapists to assimilate. Therapeutic progress thus far has been empirical, and the new information from immunology and genetics urgently needs integration into treatment programs. Pediatric oncologists also need better lines of communication with immunologists so that research can be targeted to clinical problems of importance. Thus studies are needed to help explain the frequent homing of lymphoid cells to bone marrow and meninges, while such homing occurs less frequently in the testicles. With such coordinated research, we may be able to look forward to the cure of lymphomatous diseases in children in the coming decade.

References

1. Lukes RJ, Collins RD: Immunologic characterization of human malignant lymphomas. *Cancer 34:1488–1503, 1974.*
2. Lukes RJ, Collins RD: New approaches to the classification of the lymphomata. *Br J Cancer 31(suppl. 2):1–28, 1975.*
3. Wollner N, Bruchenal JH, Lieberman PH, *et al*: Non-Hodgkin's lymphoma in children; a comparative study of two modalities of therapy. *Cancer 37:123–134, 1976.*
4. Wollner N, Jereb B: Multidisciplinary LSA2-L2 protocol treatment of non-Hodgkin's lymphoma in children; a review of 73 cases. *Proc Am Soc Clin Oncol 20:298, 1979.*
5. Gershon RK: Immune regulation; introduction. *Fed Proc 38:2051–2052, 1979.*
6. Broder S, Uchiyama T, Waldmann TA: Current concepts in immunoregulatory T-cell neoplasms. *Cancer Treat Rep 63:607–612, 1979.*
7. Toledano SR, Meadows AT: Chapter 3, this volume.
8. Ziegler JL: Chapter 8, this volume.
9. Duque L, Wollner N, Miller DR: LSA2-L2 treatment of non-Hodgkin's lymphoma (NHL) in children with partial and extensive bone marrow replacement. *Proc Am Assoc Cancer Res 20:113, 1979.*
10. deSousa M: Ecotaxis, ecotaxopathy, and lymphoid malignancy: terms, facts and predictions, in Twomey JJ, Good RA (eds): *The Immunopathology of Lymphoreticular Neoplasms. Comprehensive Immunology,* Vol. 4. Plenum, New York, 1978, pp. 325—353.
11. Hall JG, Hopkins J, Orlans E: Migration pathways of lymphoid cells with reference to the gut immunoglobulins and lymphomata. *Biochem Soc Trans. 5:1581–1583, 1977.*
12. Cantor H, Gershon RK: Immunological circuits; cellular composition. *Fed Proc 38:2058–2064, 1979.*

13. Broder S, Waldmann TA: The suppressor-cell network in cancer. (first of two parts). *N Engl J Med 299:1281–1284, 1978.*
14. Broder S, Waldmann TA: The suppressor-cell network in cancer. (second of two parts). *N Engl J Med 299:1335–1341, 1978.*
15. Broder S, Poplack D, Whang-Peng J, *et al*: Characterization of a suppressor-cell leukemia; evidence for the requirement of an interaction of two T-cells in the development of human suppressor effector cells. *N Engl J Med 298:66–72, 1978.*
16. Janeway CA: Helper T-cell interactions. *Fed Proc 38:2071–2074, 1979.*
17. Mott M: Chapter 5, this volume.

INDEX

Abdominal involvement (*see also* Bowel), 15, 50–56, 65–75, 78, 82–85, 95–103, 109–112, 117, 125, 134–137, 167
Acetazolamide (diamox), 119
Acid phosphatase activity, 25, 46–55, 153
Acidosis
  lactic, 124–125, 136
  metabolic, 120
Adriamycin, 82–86, 98, 112, 138, 160
Age incidence, 13–15, 46–58, 64, 69, 73, 132
Allopurinol, 71–75, 116–120
Antigens, 2–8, 39–58, 64–65, 74, 78, 165–171
  ALL, 38–39, 42–49, 54
  EBNA, 43, 47, 131, 142
  E-rosetting, 22–26, 31, 39–43, 46, 49–50, 54–56, 71, 74, 153
  HLA, 38, 165, 171
  HTLA, 22, 25, 38–42, 45–50, 54
  I-a like, 38, 42–43, 46–49, 55
  myeloid, 42
  nuclear, 2–3
  viral capsid, 3
Antisera, 42–43, 47, 52, 169–171
  monoclonal, 42, 48, 52
Ataxia telangiectasia, 4–5
Autoimmunity, 7–9, 169–170
  disease, 7–9
  hemolytic anemia, 7
  S.L.E., 7

B cell (*see also* Cell), 1–8, 21, 25, 31, 38, 41, 46–58, 69–71, 78–82, 131, 147–148, 156, 165–170
  follicular, 42, 56
  postfollicular, 41, 56
  neoplasm (*see* Tumor, B cell)
Beta glucuronidase, 25
Bicarbonate
  serum, 116–117
  therapy, sodium, 116, 119, 123–124, 136
Biopsy, 65–66, 73, 108–112, 116, 151
Blast cell (*see* Cell, neoplastic)
Bleomycin, 83, 138
Bloom's syndrome, 5
Bone, 27, 77, 123
  lymphoma of, 27, 69, 77–78, 101–103, 111–117, 120–125, 160
  scan, 66
Bone marrow (*see also* Leukemia), 8, 22, 38–41, 45–46, 50–56, 64–68, 69–78, 82–89, 95, 100, 109–118, 120–121, 125, 133–134, 141–143, 147–161, 166–168, 171
Bowel, 27, 46, 54, 66–71, 83–87, 96–98, 116, 121–125, 133, 147, 155–158, 161, 168

Calcitonin therapy, 123
Calcium
  serum, 116–118, 120–125, 136
  excretion, 122–123
Cancer (*see also* Tumor)
  center, Memorial Sloan-Kettering, 68–69, 75, 84, 98, 101, 108
  institute, National, 82
  institute, Sidney Farber, 85
  study group, Children's (CCSG), 64, 69, 73, 85, 98
  study group, UK Children's, 87
  Southwest Oncology Group, 82
Cell (*see also* Lymphocyte)
  B (*see* B cell)
  count, white, 25–27, 65–66, 71, 108, 111
  differentiation, 37–38, 166, 169–170
  follicular center, 28, 58, 71, 78, 166
  giant, 47
  large (histiocyte), 27, 33, 53
  lymphoid, 39, 43, 63, 76, 82, 123, 168–171
  myeloid, 39
  neoplastic (malignant), 17, 21, 26–29, 31, 58, 63–65, 70–73, 77–78, 113–118, 120–124, 131–134, 151–154, 157–158, 166–171
  null (non-T, non-B), 1, 5, 25–27, 43–48, 54–58, 75–78, 147

plasma, 38, 41–42
pre-B, 38–42, 46, 58
pre-T, 46, 50, 54, 56–58
stem, 38–39, 58, 143
T (*see* T cell)
Central nervous system, 45, 50, 64, 66–74, 77–84, 95–101, 107–108, 113–118, 125, 133–137, 141–142, 147–161, 169–171
prophylactic therapy, 84–87, 98–103, 113, 137–141, 158–161, 166–168
Cerebrospinal fluid (CSF), 45, 66, 78, 111–115, 133–134, 141, 152–154, 157
Chemotherapy (*see* Therapy)
Chromosomes (*see also* Cytogenetics), 2–5, 131
Complement, 21–31, 39–43
C3 component, 21, 25, 39–41, 46, 49–52, 54–56
Corticosteroids, 6–8, 71–74, 82, 85–86, 98, 109, 113–116, 123, 138–139, 160, 171
Creatinine, serum, 116–118
Cyclophosphamide (cytoxan), 8, 71, 82, 84–86, 98, 112, 116, 138–139, 142–143, 171
Cytochemistry, enzyme, 14, 52, 151–153
Cytogenetics (*see also* Chromosomes), 1–4
Cytology (*see also* Cell), 1, 22, 47–52, 56–58, 68, 73, 134, 151–154
Cytoplasm, 47–48
immunoglobulin, 47, 50
Cytosine arabinoside, 113, 138–139, 141–143
Cytotoxic drugs (*see* Therapy)

Dactinomycin, 96
Deoxynucleotidyl transferase (DNA), 38, 131
Diagnosis, 63–64, 69–73, 78, 83–87, 101, 107–113, 116–118, 134, 140–143, 149–151, 154–159, 167
Diphenylhydantoin, 8, 65

E rosettes (*see* Antigens)
Epidemiology, 13, 63, 131, 155–156, 161
Epipodophyllotoxins, 83
Etiology, 1–9, 117, 120, 124, 132

Folinic acid, 113

Gastrointestinal tract (*see* Bowel)
Gonads
lymphoma of, 27
ovaries, 65, 112, 133
testes, 45, 65, 73, 149, 160, 168, 171
Graft-versus-host reaction, 8

Hemoglobin, 65, 71
Histiocytosis, malignant, 37, 45, 52–58
Histopathology, 13–34, 37, 43, 47, 56–58, 63–65, 69, 73–74, 78, 81, 83, 97, 101, 117, 120, 131, 134, 148, 151, 154–158, 165–168
Rappaport classification, 14, 43, 45, 71, 74, 96, 156, 166
Lukes Collins classification, 22, 29, 71, 74, 156, 166
Kiel (Lennert) classification, 37, 43, 46
Hodgkin's disease (*see* Lymphoma, Hodgkin's)
Hypercalcemia (*see* Calcium)
Hyperkalemia (*see* Potassium)
Hyperuricemia (*see* Uric acid)

Immune response, 1, 42, 165
Immune system (*see* Lymphoreticular system)
Immunodeficiency
congenital, 1, 4–6, 8–9, 64
Bruton's hypogammaglobulinemia, 5
Immunofluorescence, 42, 65
Immunoglobulins, 6, 38, 41–43, 46–53, 71, 170
F(ab), 42
Fc fragment, 21, 39–43, 48–52, 54–56
intracytoplasmic, 31, 54
light and heavy chains, 22, 41–42, 55–56
surface, 17, 21–22, 25, 31, 38, 42–43, 47–56, 71, 131, 170
Immunotherapy, 142
Incidence (*see* Epidemiology)
Intestine (*see* Bowel)
Irradiation (*see* Therapy)

Kidney, 65, 71, 75, 98, 107, 116–117, 120–121, 125, 133–136, 169
dialysis, 120, 122, 124, 136
function, 66, 75, 117–120, 122–125, 134–136

obstruction (*see* Obstruction, renal)
stones, 117–118, 120, 123–124

Lactic dehydrogenase (LDH) serum, 116–117, 134
Laparotomy (*see* Surgery)
Leukemia
acute lymphoblastic, 5, 17, 22, 25–27, 37, 45–50, 54–58, 63–65, 67–77, 84–90, 95–96, 100, 113, 117–119, 121–124, 134, 147–161, 167, 170
acute myeloblastic, 55–56, 154
acute monocytic, 52, 147–149
bovine, 2
chronic lymphocytic, 4, 22, 41, 54, 157, 166
chronic myelocytic, 2, 4, 38
feline, 2
Liver, 65, 71, 88, 109–110, 133, 169
function, 66, 75, 124
Lymph node, 21–25, 39–43, 45–48, 50–53, 65–66, 69–78, 81–82, 96–98, 101, 109–113, 116, 133, 156, 166–169
germinal center, 31, 39, 41, 47
paracortical area (*see also* Lymphadenopathy), 25
Lymphadenopathy, 22, 45, 65, 71–73, 75–76, 82, 116, 133
immunoblastic (*see also* Lymphoproliferative disorder), 7–8
Lymphocyte, 3–6, 13, 38–41, 123, 148, 165, 168–170
B-lymphocyte (*see* B cell)
T-lymphocyte (*see* T cell)
Lymphoma (*see also* Histopathologic classification)
bovine, 2
Burkitt's, 2–3, 5–8, 14–17, 21–22, 27–29, 43, 47–48, 55–56, 63, 69–70, 78–82, 98, 102–103, 107–111, 116–118, 120–123, 131–143, 148–151, 156–161, 165–167
centroblastic, 43, 45, 48, 53
convoluted cell, 22, 26, 74, 78, 156
diffuse
lymphoblastic, 14–15, 22, 25–27, 33, 38, 43–50, 53–54, 58
poorly differentiated, 14–17, 22, 54, 71–74, 113, 151, 156
undifferentiated, non Burkitt (pleomorphic), 14–17, 27, 33, 45–47, 53–55, 58, 69, 74, 82–85, 142, 147–149, 156, 160
well differentiated, 14–15, 22, 95, 156, 166
feline, 2
histiocytic, 5–6, 14–15, 27–29, 31, 33, 45–47, 56, 64, 82, 147–149, 156–158
Hodgkin's, 13, 63–67, 76, 81–83, 95–96, 134, 166
immunoblastic, 8, 43–47, 50, 53–54, 58
nodular, 14–15, 27, 33, 37, 53–54, 78, 81, 95, 149, 156, 166
Lymphoproliferative disorder, 2, 5, 7
Lymphoreticular system, 63–64, 132, 165–171

Macrophage, 22–31
"starry sky" (*see also* Phagocyte), 17, 22, 29
Malaria, relation to lymphoma, 4, 15
Mannitol therapy, 120
Marek's disease, 2
Masses, effects of tumor, 107–116, 125
Mediastinum, 22, 25, 46–47, 50, 54–56, 64–75, 82–87, 95, 98–99, 108–109, 113, 125, 147–148, 153–161
Meninges (*see* Central nervous system)
6-Mercaptopurine, 87, 119, 138, 171
Metabolic effects, 107, 116–125
Methotrexate, 73, 84–87, 96–98, 100–101, 103, 113, 116, 138–139, 141, 160–161
Methramycin, 117, 123
Mononuclear phagocyte system, 52, 56, 170
Mononucleosis, infectious, 3

Nasopharynx, 27, 65–66, 77, 108
Neoplasm (*see* Tumor)
Neuroblastoma, 5, 13, 63, 108
Nitrogen mustard, 82
Nitrosureas, 83, 138–139, 141–143
Nucleus, 22, 26
chromatin, 22
convolutions, 22, 26, 74
membrane, 28
size, 17, 29

Obstruction
bowel, 70, 107–108, 111, 137
renal, 111, 117
respiratory, 73–75, 78, 99, 107–109, 125
superior vena caval, 73, 99, 107–109
Orbit, involvement of, 65, 77, 108, 125
Osteoclast activating factor (OAF), 121
Ovaries (*see* Gonads)

Paranasal sinuses (*see* Nasopharynx)
Parathormone, 121
Pathology (*see* Histopathology)
Pericardium, 65, 73
Peyer's patches (*see also* Bowel), 65, 169
Phenotype, features of cell, 37, 42–43, 45–47, 50, 52–58
Phosphate
serum, 116, 120–123, 125, 136
therapy, 123
Platelet count, 65, 71
Pleura, 22, 73
effusion, 22, 50, 65, 73, 75, 107, 109, 111
involvement, 47, 65, 156
Potassium, serum, 116–120, 122, 124–125, 136
Prednisone (*see* Corticosteroids)
Procarbazine, 82
Prognosis, 27, 65, 67, 69–70, 83–84, 97–98, 101, 107, 111, 134–137, 140–142, 165–166
Proptosis, 77, 108
Prostaglandins, 121
Protocol, treatment (*see also* Therapy), 64, 75, 84–87, 99, 160, 166–167

Radiotherapy (*see* Therapy, radiation)
Rappaport classification (*see* Histopathology)
Regimen (*see* Protocol)
Relapse, 71, 78, 83–84, 87, 95–96, 100–103, 133, 137, 140–143, 148, 151, 159–161
Remission, 73, 87, 98–99, 125, 134, 139–143
Retinoblastoma, 13, 16
Rhabodomyosarcoma, embryonal, 13, 16
Roentgenography
barium series, 66, 71, 111
chest, 66–67, 71, 74–75, 111
intravenous pyelography, 66, 71, 75, 116, 118
lymphangiography, 67, 110–111
myelography, 113, 115
skeletal, 66, 113, 116
tomography, 66–67, 110–111

Sarcomas, 13
bone, 13
immunoblastic (*see* Lymphoma, immunoblastic)
reticulum cell (*see* Lymphoma, histiocytic)
round cell, 15
Steinberg (*see* Lymphoma, lymphoblastic)
Sex ratio, 13, 44, 48–50, 64, 69, 73, 77
Site of involvement (*see also individual sites*), 64–65, 100, 107, 134
Skeletal system (*see* Bone)
Skin, involvement of, 65, 78, 168
Spinal cord (*see* Central nervous system)
Spleen, 27, 41, 65, 69–71, 133, 168–169
Staging
classification, 67–69, 83, 98, 166–168
clinical, 63, 65–67, 77, 84, 86–87, 98–100, 107–109, 133, 136, 140–143, 149–151, 154–156, 158–160, 170
laparotomy, 67, 83
Surgery (*see also* Staging), 67, 78, 82–85, 90, 96–98, 103, 108–112, 116, 125, 136–137, 140–142, 158
Survival pattern (*see also* Prognosis), 75, 78, 82–87, 95–96, 98–101, 107, 137, 141, 154, 159, 161

T cell (*see also* Cell), 1–8, 22, 25–27, 38–43, 45–50, 53–58, 65, 71, 74, 78, 82, 90, 159, 165–171
cytotoxic, 3, 169–170
fetal, 41
helper, 169–171
marker, 1, 31
neoplasm, 2, 39–59, 82, 147–148, 153–159, 166–167
prethymic, 38, 45
postthymic, 39
suppressor, 7, 22, 38–39, 169–171
Terminal deoxynucleotidyl transferase (Tdt), 25, 38–39, 43–46, 48–50, 54–55, 74, 147
Testes (*see* Gonads)
Therapeutic ratio (*see also* Toxicity), 83

Therapy, 70, 78, 81, 95–96, 100, 113, 116–117, 122, 125, 136–143, 149, 155, 159–160, 165–171
  chemotherapy, 8, 27, 70–71, 75, 78, 81–91, 96, 98–100, 107–117, 119, 123–125, 136–143, 149, 155, 159–160, 165–171
  immunosuppressive, 6–7, 83
  induction, 84, 139–141
  irradiation, 70, 76, 78, 82, 90, 95–103, 107–109, 111–117, 125, 137–142, 159–161, 169–171
  maintenance, 84, 87, 139, 160
  prophylactic (*see* Central nervous system)
  surgical (*see* Surgery)
Thymoma, 56
Thymus (*see also* Mediastinum), 7, 37, 39, 45, 58, 66, 74, 148, 169
Thyroid, 65, 108
Toxicity of therapy (*see also* Therapy), 85, 96–98, 100–103, 119
Transplantation, 6–7
  bone marrow, 8
  renal, 8, 64
  thymic, 7
Tumor, 3–5, 8, 64, 81–83, 98, 108–113, 117–118, 122, 125, 133–137, 139–143, 165–171
  B cell, 4, 8, 52–54
  CNS, 5, 13
  facial, 15, 116, 132–133
  lymphoreticular, 5
  lysis syndrome, acute, 124, 135–136, 142
  monoclonal, 4, 131
  plasma cell, 8
  Wilms' (*see also* Lymphoma), 5, 13, 63

Ultrasonography, 6, 111
Urea nitrogen, 7, 111, 116–118, 121
Uric acid, 65–66, 71, 116–120, 122–125, 136

Vincristine (Oncovin), 8, 71, 82, 85–86, 98, 113, 116, 138–139, 160
Virus, 1–3, 132
  DNA, 2–3
  EB, 2–8, 15–16, 69, 131–133, 142, 165
  endogenous, 2
  exogenous, 2
  genome, 2–3
  herpes-type, 2, 16
  oncogenic, 4–9
  RNA, type C, 1–2

Waldeyer's ring, 65, 96, 98, 108
Wilms' tumor (*see* Tumor)
Wiskott-Aldrich syndrome, 4

Xanthine, 117, 119–120, 125
X-ray (*see* Roentgenography)